A self-help book that makes you

SLEEP BETTER

FEEL BETTER

LIVE BETTER

By ANA KAWAI

SLEEP BETTER FEEL BETTER LIVE BETTER

Edited by
ANA KAWAI
63630 Saint Germain L'herm

Legal deposit: August 2020
First Edition

Printed on demand via Amazon
ISBN **9798661245120**

Copyright © 2020 by Ana Kawai
All right reserved, including the right of reproduction in whole or in part in any form.

Cover by ANA KAWAI

TABLE OF CONTENTS

FOREWORD

CHAPTER 1: WHAT YOU CAN EXPECT

CHAPTER 2: THE POWER OF A GOOD NIGHT'S SLEEP
I. General Information
II. Why Sleeping Well Is So Important

CHAPTER 3: THE KEYS TO MEETING MR SANDMAN
THE 6 PRECIOUS STONES
I. Motivation
II. Awareness Of The Situation
III. Taking Action
IV. Understanding
V. 'Switch Button'
VI. Strategy- Last Precious Stone

CHAPTER 4: SELF-ASSESSMENT
I. Sleep Pattern Tool - Id Cards
II. Current Situation Tool – Analyse

CHAPTER 5: BASICS AND HABITS
I. Holistic Approach Of Your Body
II. Atmosphere And Sleep
III. Magnetic Fields
IV. Listen To Your Body
V. Shower And Sleep
VI. Sport And Sleep
VII. 'Protect' Your Brain
VIII. Circadian Rhythm And Sleep

CHAPTER 6: YOUR ANCHOR FOR LIFE
I. General Information
II. Breathing Techniques
III. 10 Day Challenge Breathing Exercise

CHAPTER 7: THE ART OF LAUGHING
I. Why is laughing so good
II. Sleep disorders and laughter therapy
III. What about Smiling
IV. Everyday Challenge - Laugh Checklist

CHAPTER 8: GRATITUDE
I. Introduction To Gratitude
II. What Does A Gratitude Journal Look Like
III. Power Of Gratitude On Our Brain
IV. 21 Day Challenge Gratitude Journal
V. Gratitude Letter

CHAPTER 9: POSITIVE MINDSET
I. Neuroscience And Inner Strength
II. How Can You Change Your Mindset
III. How To Shift Your Mindset To A Positive One
IV. Bad Day Positive Challenge
V. Daily Positive Mindset Checklist

CHAPTER 10: PLAN TOMORROW
I. 1000 Reasons To Plan Your Day
II. What To Do And What To Write
III. Plan Tomorrow Checklist

CHAPTER 11: MUSIC - THE CONDUCTOR OF YOUR NIGHT
I. General Information
II. Water And Brainwave Facts
III. When To Listen

CHAPTER 12: THE POWER OF NATURE
I. Natural Remedies Vs Traditional Medicine
II. Natural Tips That Enhance A Better Sleep
III. Crystals
IV. The Power Of Animals

CHAPTER 13: MEDITATION
I. General Information
II. Meditation And' Meditation'
III. Meditation And Health
IV. Neuroscience And Meditation
V. How To Meditate
VI. Meditation Practices

CHAPTER 14: DREAMS
I. The Science Of Dreams
II. What Can We Do About Our Dreams

Chapter 15: THE BEAUTY OF REIKI
I. General Information
II. How Does It Work
III. Benefits Of Reiki
IV. More Than A Spiritual Practice

CHAPTER 16: OSTEOPATHY
I. Osteopathy For Dummies
II. The Benefits Of Osteopathy
III. How Osteopathy Helps You Sleep
IV. What Happens During A Treatment
V. Your Responsibility

CONCLUSION
INDEX
ACKNOWLEDGTEMENTS
BIBLIOGRAPHY

Sleep Better, Feel Better, Live Better.

FOREWORD

Five years ago, I decided to leave my birth country to travel for a year which became a four-year journey.

I graduated in osteopathy a year before I left. This moment of my life wasn't the best one. I believed that I was 'cursed' and that no matter how hard I tried to improve my situation, I would never be happy. I was depressed.
For many years I suffered from insomnia. I had terrible nightmares and would wake up tired, anxious and often bored with my life. The only good night's sleep I had was after a good rock climbing session with my friends or a day of snowboarding.

One of my dreams was to go to New Zealand. I didn't know why yet but I had to leave France and travel overseas. I wanted to step outside of this negative bubble I had been trapped in for my entire life. New Zealand felt like a natural therapy for me. I found more peace in my sleep and had less nightmares and insomnia. I know now these good results were due to the new environment I was living in, the vibes of the country and its people. I then travelled to Australia and the quality of my sleep started to worsen again. I was so busy dealing with certain troubles that I forgot about myself. I underestimated how important it is to sleep well and how much things are interconnected.

I had been living in different countries and experienced all sorts of things. You can go through stressful situations on a higher frequency than when you live in your comfortable 'home sweet home'. Sleeping well can be a big challenge, sometimes. Travelling is enriching and exhausting at the same time and this is why it is so important to sleep well. You need good vibes upon wakening and enough energy-resources to deal with frequent or unexpected events.

A few years of travels and meeting all sorts of personalities changed my perception of life and helped me improve my well-being including my sleep pattern. As well, I initiated myself to Reiki healing because I was convinced it would help me feel better. And it did.

I wrote about how to improve people's quality of sleep and life for many reasons. Firstly, sharing what I learnt and experienced was a good way to reinforce my knowledge on the topic and consolidate my new habits. Secondly, everything being interconnected, learning more about myself was a way to learn more about others therefore share more. Last but not least, if it worked for me, it might work for you. Sleep disorders are such an epidemic in the world that if my book can be of any help, I would be so happy and grateful to be one of those who can make a positive difference in your life.

This book is based on my personal experience, my studies, a lot of reflective work and a desire to share. I gathered information from all around the world, from experts in the field, books, podcasts, and some wise advice from friends and people I met on the road…

What works for me may not be what you're looking for but I'm sure it will bring some positivity in your life if this is what you're genuinely looking for. Even if only a fraction of you tries to apply what I suggest, it is already a success. So, thank you in advance.
I sincerely wish my perception of life will enlighten some of you, guide you, and support you in your attempts to sleep better, feel better, and live better.

"We find what we expect to find, and we receive what we ask for."

ELBERT HUBBARD

CHAPTER 1
WHAT YOU CAN EXPECT

Before going any further, I must inform you that I am a certified osteopath and a Reiki practitioner passionate about self-development, however this book is under no circumstances a substitute for medical advice. If you have a health condition or believe you may have one, please refer to your general practitioner who, I am sure, will be delighted to guide you towards a treatment adapted to your needs.

With this book, you are embarking on a journey designed to help you figure out how to improve the quality of your sleep, how to feel better and live better. It involves natural methods and concepts that I have learnt from people, developed on my own and what I have been using for years. They supported me in my quest to 'spend more time' with Mr Sandman; you know, this mythical character who sprinkles magical sand onto your eyes to make you sleep and have beautiful dreams!

This book provides you with information, stories or facts you may already know. However, keep in mind that refreshing your memory is a good thing and can make you use your knowledge in a different way that can benefit you. You can expect minor or radical changes in your life and in the way you think. If you get up tired every morning or often feel that you are not in the mood because you had a bad night, you can expect positive changes. You may have less nightmares and ease the negative emotions related to them.

If you hibernate as long as a bear does and still feel exhausted every morning, this book, with your active participation of course, may help you experience more restorative nights and reduce your need to 'oversleep'. You can expect changes if you hit the snooze button every five minutes, preferring not to go to work than earning money, or if you snore as loud as an old steam train preventing your partner from sleeping.
Does this sound like you?

If you are a newbie in self-improvement, this is perfectly fine because all you need to know is to read, be willing to try, act, and enjoy the results. I believe you will discover simple and very interesting ways to change or adopt new habits that will improve your well-being.

***

This book is an honest experience and may challenge you. The real deal may be to turn your old habits into new ones supposed to help you feel better. You have to sign a new contract with yourself that says,

'I am ready to sleep better, feel better, live better, and I understand that it is my responsibility to make it happen'.

HOW TO GET THE MOST FROM THIS BOOK

First of all, I won't be offended if you decide to let this book sit in your toilet (as long as you don't use it for another purpose than reading it).
You should take your time and study the book. Each detail can be the answer you're looking for. It's not a competition.
This book landed in your hands for a reason. Get your favourite pen and paper and get ready to do the 'homework' I have prepared for you. Work thoroughly on the chapters and sentences that catch and require your attention. You will easily recognize them.

WHAT YOU CAN EXPECT

They may inspire you or trigger unpleasant emotions such as, *'No way I'm not doing this!'*, *'I disagree'*, *'I don't have time'*, or the famous, *'I already know that'*. You sometimes think you know, but you don't always know, and you may not know that you don't know. I'll let you consider that...

You might start reading this book with a sceptical mind or negative thoughts like the ones I had a few years ago. It's okay, just acknowledge what you feel and keep reading anyway. Even if you don't understand everything, be open-minded and if you firmly believe that this book will help you sleep better or improve an aspect or situation in your life, it will most likely be the case.

Once you read this book, go through the end of each chapter (*In a nutshell*) one more time to keep the key elements in mind. Try at least one of the challenges every one or two weeks and write down your experience to keep track of your progress.

I sincerely hope this book will make a positive difference in your life and bring a smile to your face.

Happy reading!

IN A NUTSHELL

- This book is not a substitute for medical advice. You are encouraged to refer to your doctor if you have, or believe you may have a condition.

- You can expect minor to radical changes in your life and the way you think.

- Results depend on your willingness to participate with me on this journey.

- It all starts with a new contract you sign with and for yourself,
'I am ready to sleep better, feel better, live better, and I understand that it is my responsibility to make it happen'.

- To get the most from this book, you should work thoroughly on what caught your attention using the different exercises or concepts related to the topic.

- You should put aside any sceptical or negative thoughts and firmly believe that you can make a change that benefits your sleep, your feelings, and your emotions.

"A well spent day brings Happy Sleep".
LEONARDO DAVINCI

CHAPTER 2
THE POWER OF A GOOD NIGHT'S SLEEP

I. GENERAL INFORMATION

The average worldwide sleeping time is between six and eight hours per night. If you sleep seven hours a night and live until the age of 75, you will spend about 20 000 hours sleeping.
That is thirty years or close to one-third of your life spent in bed. Wow! You deserve to treat yourself to a good mattress!

With these numbers, you understand now that improving the quality of your sleep can potentially make a big difference to your life.

Sleep disorders are a real public health epidemic. Our quality of sleep is underestimated, although it is one of the most important aspects of our lives. Restless leg syndrome*, insomnia, circadian rhythm* troubles (chapter 5), snoring and sleep apnoea are amongst the main common sleep disorders people suffer from. This kind of disorder can trigger symptoms such as headaches, aching muscles, excessive sleepiness, daytime somnolence and many other health issues. In the long term, it can lead to depression, lack of interest in life, trouble focusing on anything, isolation or even a severe lack of confidence because you cannot think clearly and start doubting all the decisions you take in life, etc.

The good news is that it is never too late to do something about it. It is only too late when you have both feet in the grave.

***

In Australia, the Health Sleep Foundation's Annual Report 2018 reveals that inadequate sleep is highly prevalent and affects 4 out of 10 Australian adults. (1)

In New Zealand, a research conducted for Sovereign 2015 based on a sample of 1600 kiwis, counts one-third of them as suffering from a sleep disorder. (2)

In the United-States, the studies led by the American Sleep apnoea Association show that 50 to 70 million Americans of all ages, struggle with the quality of their sleep. (3)

In France, the INSV/MGEN in 2015 concludes that 73% of the population complains about sleep disorders and at least 42 % suffer from four of the main common sleep disorders previously mentioned. (4)

Finally, in the U.K, it is estimated that one third of the population suffers from insomnia, which is about 200,000 working days 'of wasted money' per year. (5)

Another alarming fact is the amount of people relying on tablets to fall asleep or sleep. A government survey led in 2013 showed that 4% of Americans use sleeping pills. This percentage only refers to the tablets people can obtain with prescription and doesn't take into account the amount of people taking illegal drugs. (6)

II. WHY SLEEPING WELL IS SO IMPORTANT

WHAT HAPPENS DURING THE NIGHT

A good night's sleep is essential for your body as it helps you regain the energy you have expended during the day. It is all the more important if you live a 'hectic life'. (6)

Sleep is divided into several stages in which important physiological reactions happen to allow your body and your mind to rest. They help you regain the necessary energy you will need for the following day. Wihtout adequate and uninterrupted nights, your body doesn't have the chance to fully complet these stages and you will experience the symptoms of sleep deprivation. [5] Besides, it may increase your 'risk of obesity, heart disease and diabetes, and can lead to shortened life expectancy'. The time needed to recover from unrestul nights tends to increase with age and is dependant on the status of your health. The body doesn't repair itself as quickly as when you are young. It works the same way for hangovers (I'm sure you can relate to that!). It lasts zero to a few hours when you're 18 years old and may take a whole day when you are 40 years old.

SCIENCE CORNER

Your night runs through a succession of stages that are made up of two cycles (or two parts) in a main cycle: the Non-Rapid Eye movement or NREM cycle, and the Rapid Eye Movement or REM cycle. The main cycle lasts about 90 minutes and keeps repeating itself all night with certain variations. [7]

Each cycle is characterized by a process of brain waves activity.
To communicate together and fulfil their mission or function, the cells of the brain need to synchronize at specific amplitudes and frequencies which form the brainwaves.

The first part or first cycle, NREM represents ¾ of your night and is composed of four stages.

Stage one. It is the lightest and shortest one and is supposed to last about ten minutes. It is when you feel drowsy. It is the stage people have the most trouble with because they don't manage to disconnect (overthinking, physical pain, etc.).
This is the stage of the alpha waves.

IN A NUTSHELL

- You sleep one-third of your life (about 30 years).

- Sleep disorders can take many forms and are more frequent than what we think.

- Sleep covers a succession of mechanisms that are vital to maintain a good body homeostasis.

- The night is made of five stages that repeat themselves about every 90 minutes.

- Each stage is defined by certain brainwaves that are activity-related.

- The stages 3, 4, and 5 are the most restorative ones.

- Interrupting a stage can cause light to severe symptoms.

Your dreams occur during the last quarter of your night called REM sleep.

"Rowing harder doesn't help if the boat is headed in the wrong direction."
KENICHI OHMAE

CHAPTER 3
KEYS TO MEETING MR SANDMAN

Changing a situation requires more than a simple wish.
It is a commitment.

A lot of self-development books that I read were highly enriching and fascinating, but most of the time I thought something important was missing. Reading is a first step to growing and empowering oneself but if you don't understand or don't know what to do next, the chances of getting results are very low. The books that helped me were the ones that encouraged me to act.

Reaching a good balance in your life and improving the quality of your sleep requires you to question yourself and be active.
Keep in mind that a self-development book is meant to support you and not to endorse your responsibilities.

The keys to meeting Mr Sandman are a combination of methods or tools, advice and concepts which are designed to help you get more results while studying this book. They are based on a holistic approach to the body, the brain and the mind.
I call them 'the precious stones'. It has nothing to do with 'my precious' ring in the Lord of the Rings movie even though sleeping better could make you live longer. I have been using many precious stones for years and decided to make use of them in this book.

If you are willing to sleep better, feel better and live better, you need to pay attention to some details (precious stones) that may seem irrelevant initially, but are in fact essential to making a significant difference.

The concept is to challenge your ability to question yourself.
The introspection work, exercises and challenges you go through in this book are meant to make you see your life from another perspective.

THE 6 PRECIOUS STONES
I. MOTIVATION

Motivation is the first precious stone you need to drop in your bucket. It is a skill you need to develop to get things done. It is what drives you to persevere with something until the end.

IDENTIFYING THE 'DANGERS' TO STAY MOTIVATED

Impatience, lack of faith, fatigue, negative attitude or stress are the kind of dangers that can reduce your motivation when you want to change your old habits for new ones.
These habits can be part of your system of beliefs or part of your old routine (diet, physical exercise, work, hobbies, etc.).

When we start something new that is supposed to be good for us, 'human nature' usually takes control of the situation. We start finding excuses such as *'I am too tired to do this now, I'll try tomorrow, what I try never works anyway, it's a waste of time, etc.'* The main reason for this behaviour is because 'we believe' that these dangers are too strong and/or because the motivation to achieve our goal(s) is too weak to keep us on track. Unless you had a busy and productive day, these excuses are conscious or unconscious justifications you find for not doing what needs to be done. They lead to procrastination. Lack of motivation always leads to procrastination. Sounds familiar?
Let's get started!

🖉 *Take a pen and paper and answer this question quickly. The first number you think of is a good one because it comes without interference (overthinking). On a scale of 0 to 10, 10 being a lot, how much do you procrastinate?*

Procrastination may happen anytime during this journey when I give you some exercises, challenges or most likely during the introspection work in the next chapter. It can simply happen by not answering this first question because you can't be bothered to stand up and grab a pen and paper. But, I'm sure you played the game...

ABOUT THE NATURAL TENDENCY OF THE BRAIN

If you suffer from sleep disorders, it is obviously for a reason.
No matter what the cause is, you have to change certain aspects of your life to get results. You need to change your behaviour facing the kind of dangers we mentioned and which leads to procrastination/being passive.

The problem is that we generally start doing things, make resolutions, and as time passes by, we lose track of the original reasons that pushed us to make that change. It is a natural rule. We are trapped in our everyday life and hassles instead of focusing on things that could be important. We are 'busy enough' and it would be too much to add an extra task to our already busy schedule.

Fact: This natural tendency is hard to escape because our brain is the laziest companion we have to survive. [1] The primitive hought of our brain is, 'if I survived until today this way, why would I make a change?'
Your brain creates anything possible to push you away from something you are not used to. Making a difference means you have to change something and make an effort. Your brain 'doesn't like' making efforts and 'doesn't care' if it makes you

happy as long as the primitive functions of your body are maintained.

For example, if you suffer from sleep deprivation, you don't sleep enough, but on the other hand, you keep playing video games every night when it's bedtime. To summarize, you keep wasting time everyday instead of spending valuable time with your kids, partner, or doing something that could benefit you (sleeping more, meditating, reading, etc.). You probably don't even think about your behaviour because it has become a habit. Even if this habit doesn't help you, there is no reason why your brain 'would bother' making an effort and 'help you' change your behaviour because you have survived this way until today and 'this is all that matters.'

The excuses your brain finds are endless and strengthen the bad habits that don't lead anywhere. This is why they are dangerous. They make you waste time, procrastinate, and push you to keep doing what you do and that doesn't make you feel good in the long term. These excuses can be very peculiar and disguised as lies, denials, diseases or even physical accidents. If you keep telling yourself that you won't succeed an exam, you won't succeed! Don't worry! Your conscious and unconscious mind will find a way to make you fail, and you may be sick during the exam, or have a car crash, or anything that can comfort your failure to happen. Learning how to bypass or reduce this self-sabotage brain tendency will create a much healthier environment in your life that will benefit you.

HOW TO BYPASS THE NATURAL TENDENCY OF THE BRAIN

Avoiding unnecessary obstacles and staying motivated will help you consolidate the new habits you have adopted to sleep better. How does it work?
The best way I found is to find appealing ways to reach your targets instead of forcing yourself to do too many things that you don't like or which may be too challenging at first.

For example, if you decided to run the marathon, don't try achieving the 42 kilometres distance in two weeks. Instead, take your time, set your goal, and make your step by step plan until you make it happen. To put your plan into action, it has to be strong enough to bypass your bad habits, beliefs or feelings.

I like to use images to understand certain situations better.
If you think about hamsters in their cage, they are 'programmed' to run in a wheel all day, eat, run, eat, sleep, etc., and don't even know why, probably.
The human version is similar in that we mostly wake up, eat, work, eat, work, eat, and sleep, etc. Also, the most common human mind-set in life is to complain about problems without trying to find a real solution. We are often trapped in a loop with our old habits and beliefs. You must work on this 'cheeky' weakness (tendency to procrastinate) to reach your goals
and stop acting like victims.

Let's go back to hamsters! If you put a glass of red wine in their cage they probably won't stop doing their activity to go and have a sip of it. But, if you put some delicious cheese and add an obstacle in their way such as water or a cat, they will remember how awesome it is to eat cheese and won't focus on their fear (water, cat). The smell is so good that they will jump out of their wheel and swim, or find a strategy to avoid the cat and fully bite into this tasty cheddar! Yum!
The 'temptation' or target (love for cheese-eat) was strong enough to bypass the natural tendency of their brain (habit to run without purpose, fear of water/cat) and bigger than a useless target (wine). The amazing feeling of love for cheese and the pleasure of its taste helped overcome all the difficulties.

Therefore, avoiding procrastination with bypassing methods will help you sleep and feel better. It will allow you to focus on your target which is improving your sleep, your health and everything else related to it, rather than on your problems.

The good news is that you are not a hamster (of course), your brain is bigger, you have more resources, and you might not need some cheese to stop procrastinating...
So, step out of your bubble!

LEARN HOW TO ENGAGE

You can find the way to bypass dangers by asking yourself the right questions. It is that simple. Ask yourself why you want to sleep better or feel better about a certain situation. We often take simple or obvious things for granted and forget about their importance.

I started and completed this book thanks to a simple but powerful combination of tools that I customized. I used the following methods to find answers and raise motivation while trying to achieve specific goals. (2). You may use it for your situation.

FIRST WAY
1) FIND A MEANINGFUL POSITIVE REASON

You need to find the initial cause or the meaningful positive reason why you want to change your habits and way to think. Having a reason to do something is a guideline.
A donkey will be more motivated to walk with a carrot in front of his face, and you won't go to work without being paid, unless you already have all the money you need and that you are passionate about your job.

✏ *Take a pen and paper and write down what you want, why, and the meaningful reason behind it.*

Example: I want to sleep better because I suffer from daily somnolence and I can't stay focused on my courses at school.

MEANINGFUL REASON: improving the quality of my health and my concentration at school.

✏ *I want (to sleep better) ... because...*

🖊 My meaningful positive reason is ...

2) FIND A POSITIVE DRIVING EMOTION

Ask yourself why the meaningful reason you just found matters. Do it until you find the emotion that can drive you to act and never give up. This emotion has to be strong enough to keep you on track until you reach your goal (like the hamster and its love for cheese).

🖊 Why does it matter that...? Why do I care about...? Why is it important?
🖊 Because ...

<u>Same example</u>: Why does it matter that I stop feeling tired all day? Why is it important to stay focused at school?
Because I think my memory would improve and it would help me have better results at school.

Keep asking yourself **'why'** until you find the emotion that counts. You will feel it.
Why do I really care about having good results at school or improving my memory?
Because I want to finish my schooling and I need good results to enter the University where I want to study.
Why does it matter? What would it mean to have all this? What it would feel like to have all this?
I would be so happy to study what I love at last. And I would feel so proud to tell my family about it.

DRIVING EMOTION: happiness to study one's passion and to share this achievement with important people.

🖊 Why do I really care about...? Because ...
🖊 Why does it matter that ...? Because...
🖊 What would that mean to have ...? What it would feel like to have...? Because...

🖉 *My positive driving emotion is...*

Take a few minutes to write down your thoughts. Consider asking a friend to help you. Friends usually see the whole picture better than we do and make us assess the situation with more objectivity. Once you identified the reason(s) and emotion(s) that matter for you, repeat them out loud or write them down on paper every day to focus on what you want. This repetition process will increase your chance of succeeding.

SECOND WAY

'Moving away' from what you don't want can be another option as well. Although, the intention you set in this case is based on a negative feeling you want to avoid, and not on a positive emotion The first option will be more robust because you will build something new based on positive thoughts that is to say a solid basis. On the contrary, hurtful triggers can control your behaviour because they correspond to unhealed emotions you don't want to experience again.

With that being said, it is still better to act than not doing anything at all. This is why considering this option can be another alternative. [4]

🖉 *I want to move away from ... because ...*

🖉 *Start to draw the following PYRAMID. It is a tool that summarizes your journey and will help you keep in mind your goals. Place it on the fridge or somewhere you go everyday.*

SLEEP BETTER
FEEL BETTER
LIVE BETTER

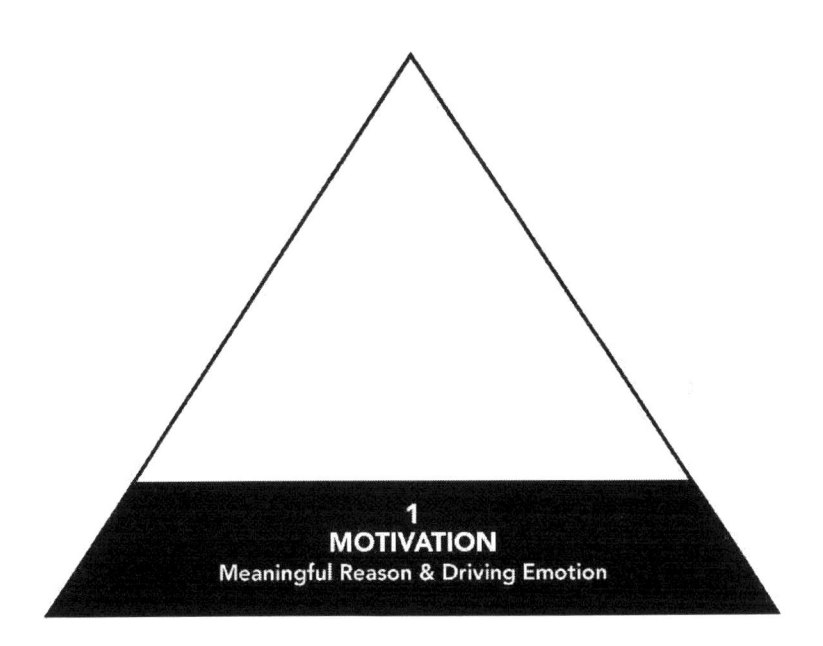

```
        /\
       /  \
      /    \
     /      \
    /        \
   /          \
  /            \
 /_____\
|        1       |
|   MOTIVATION   |
|Meaningful Reason & Driving Emotion|
```

II. AWARENESS OF THE SITUATION

The second precious stone you need to collect is about self-awareness. You need to acknowledge your situation. Knowing what is happening in your life is essential to make things work and start on a solid basis. Matt Barnett's, NLP practitioner*, develops the fundamental keys to achieving goals in one of his classes. He explains that you need to 'specify your present situation'. [3]

Your current situation corresponds to the main events occurring in your life, to your behaviour, your emotions, your beliefs, your strengths and weaknesses.

2. THE PRIORITY IS YOU

You need to make changes for you and you alone even if your decision involves someone else.

Example: Changing your habits shouldn't be because you disturb your partner's sleep but because it will improve the quality of your sleep.

You don't quit smoking for someone else but you do it to improve your health. How many people stop smoking 'for their partner' and start again after breaking up? A lot. It is mostly because their initial reason and motivation weren't strong enough.
People surrounding you may be part of a meaningful reason to make changes in your life but keep in mind that good health is the starting point for everything.

3. TIME

Time is energy. It is like refuelling your car. You are the car and the time you have is the petrol. You have a certain amount of petrol which reduces regardless of the direction you take. It is used and is not replenished without your help.
Sounds logical?
You need to use your time smartly. Over thinking or allowing your family, education or principles to prevent you from acting are a waste of time.

If running 20 minutes every morning makes you feel good,
just do it!
You will always find excuses to make no effort for things that don't count enough in your life, as much as you will always find a way to obtain what you really want.

Don't wait ten more years to change your habits to see if something good could have happened. The only moment you have and can control is now, so act today to avoid regret.

Action is key to achieving your goals. There are no results without action.

There is no action without someone to act, and you are responsible for your life. So do what needs to be done to get what you want. The countdown has already begun...

✎ Write down in your pyramid: '3. Taking action': I am responsible for my happiness. I am the priority. My power is to act now'.

IV. UNDERSTANDING

Knowing yourself is the first step to feel better. It is your power of observation that will tell you what you do wrong or right and that will make you take better decisions.

> *"Who looks outside, dreams; who looks inside, awakes."*
> CARL JUNG

If I ask you to help me and do something you've never done which requires some skills you don't have, three scenarios may happen. You may ask me to find someone else to do it or tell me you're too busy even if you may not be. The second option is that you may not help me because you don't have the knowledge to do it. The third option can be that you will do it but very badly unless you're a genius. If I now explain how to do this task, you will do it, may enjoy doing it and even do a good job.

It works the same way with your mind. If you understand your behaviour, your strengths and weaknesses, you will have better results because you know what you need to achieve your goals. Knowing the mechanism of things makes it easier because you use your logical mind to recreate the same kind of situations that have previously benefited you (strengths). As you gain experience in doing certain tasks or think a certain way, you can avoid making the same mistakes (weaknesses).

Acting with a certain common sense that you will have learnt (new beliefs, habits) will help you focus on the process and the outcome you desire instead of the difficulties that lead to procrastination. Eventually, you may be more productive.

The purpose of the next chapter is to develop the understanding you have about your situation after identifying the situation itself and your behaviour (awareness).
Understanding yourself is a must to be clear in your mind and in your intentions.

✎ Write down '4. Understanding' in your pyramid and on top of 3. Taking action.

V. 'SWITCH BUTTON'

The concept of the switch button is to let go of the 'old' to be replaced by new habits, beliefs and positive emotions. It is the fifth precious stone and key point you need to work on.

1. 'SPRING CLEANING'

Whatever causes your sleep disorders, a **spring cleaning** is essential to help you see clearly and incorporate new information better. It is easier to build a house on hard ground than on mud! What you should 'clean'/cleanse are the negative emotions (stress, anger, guilt, etc.) and beliefs that don't benefit you, or anything that leads to over thinking. These negatives tend to make you procrastinate therefore waste the time you need for action (third precious stone).

Understand the importance of this emotional spring cleaning

When a computer is full of spam and not updated it works slowly and any additional software can't load properly because there is insufficient space. It works more or less the same way with our brain; toxic thoughts or emotions can lead to non-action.
Releasing 'paralysing' emotions is a must before moving to the next step (e.g. learning new habits).

You may not be able to release the emotions of an entire life in one day but as you work progressively on them you will start feeling better.

Unbalanced emotions tend to intoxicate our minds (over thinking) and can take over our biological need to sleep (hormone imbalance). I'm sure you can remember one of those days when you try to fall asleep after a 'fight' with one of your family. Unless you're thoughtless or easily detach from arguments, it can become a hard thing to do.
It works the same way with old emotions you weren't ready to deal with from the past. Certain events can happen and trigger unhealed emotions which can be stressful.

Emotions can guide you but they shouldn't control your life. Being able to control the side effects of an emotion brings you more peace of mind and allows you to be more objective and efficient in your actions.

Find and let go of toxic emotions.

Here is one of the methods you can use to set emotions free but keep in mind there are hundreds of ways to do it as long as what you choose works for you. I came up with the following questions thanks to the experience I've had with my patients, relatives, and other people I've met on my journey. They have helped me identify, understand and release intense and past emotions.

🖋 *Take your pen and paper and answer the following questions.*

SPRING CLEANING QUESTIONS

Choose a negative emotion you feel on a recurrent basis or a recent emotion that disturbs you.
1. What does this emotion make you feel like?
2. Why does this emotion make you feel this way?
3. Do you enjoy feeling this way?

4. Why do you keep feeling this way?
5. What does feeling this way bring into your life?
6. When was the first time you felt this emotion or something similar to it?
7. What do you do to feel better? How does this emotion go away?
8. Do you always behave the same way when faced with this emotion?
9. What is the emotion trigger?
10. What can you do about it?

Ask yourself these questions as many times as you need until you find the real 'trigger' emotion, the tender point you need to set free in order to feel better. With practice you will feel more comfortable finding the solution.

A recurrent negative emotion needs to 'go away'. Your job is to 'accept' that this emotion exists, to feel it and forgive yourself and everybody/everything related to it.

You need to accept 'it' happened even if it wasn't acceptable to take responsibility for the situation. From that point onwards you can let go of any emotion that doesn't help you because you don't need it anymore.

✎ Write down on paper
I accept that I feel…
I understand why I feel this way. I feel this way because …
Thank you for experiencing this …… (feeling).
I understand that I don't need to feel …. anymore.

✎ Replace this emotion by its opposite feeling
From now on, I feel …. because (positive reason)…

It is helpful to combine these questions and affirmations with other methods to harmonise the physical, spiritual and emotional plans. The Little Stick Figures technique*, EFT techniques*, Ho'oponopono* prayer, sophrology, hypnosis and many other techniques are excellent to practise – to name a few.

2. OLD HABITS AND BELIEFS THAT DON'T BENEFIT YOU.
Understand the importance of dealing with your 'paradigms'

On top of the emotions you need to work on, are your old habits, beliefs and patterns that are called 'paradigms'. Bob Proctor, writer, teacher, motivational speaker, and Chairman and Co-Founder of Proctor Gallagher Institute, explains paradigms in his work 'Understanding the Power of Paradigm'. [5] He says that '[p]aradigms are a multitude of habits that guide every move you make'. They can control your life.

They can control your behaviour. Your old patterns and habits come from your external environment. They correspond to a massive amount of data that your brain absorbed on conscious and subconscious levels and which sculpted the way you are, the way you think, the way you feel, and the way you act.

Geek fact: 'your brain receives 400 Billion bits of information a second and we are only aware of only 2,000 of those' according to Dr. Joseph Dispenza, D.C [6]. So, imagine the whopping amount of work your brain is capable of!

It would be really hard to start something new and do it the right way if you have certain beliefs that 'hold you back'.

Here are some examples of paradigms – to name a few.

-*Girls are more fragile than boys*. This belief leads parents to overprotect their girl, give more freedom to their brother if they have one, and eventually create a feeling of injustice.
-*You cannot have everything you want in life.* This belief can lead to self-sabotaging behaviours.

4. <u>Who</u> is (was) there when you 'experience(d)' this paradigm?
5. How did you react the first time when faced with this situation? How do you react now?
6. <u>Why</u> do you keep this paradigm in mind and does it benefit you?

Shift your paradigms. Switch the button. (7)

Why change a paradigm

The way you think or behave doesn't give you the results you expect which means that you need to change something to obtain different results. Acting and thinking differently will give you different results. It is a mathematic principle.

> "If you want something you've never had, you have to do something you've never done." (8)
> JIM KWIK

According to Bob Proctor, there are only two ways to shift a paradigm. The first one is a trauma. An emotional event in your life can be powerful enough to change some of your deepest beliefs or habits and give you a good kick in the butt to change your life.

The second one is learning valuable information and repeating it until it becomes a habit or your way of thinking.

'The more you impress the image into your subconscious mind, the stronger it becomes. Eventually, the old image weakens and the new one replaces it'. (9)

You need to 'suggest' other options to your brain. You have to shift your old paradigm with a new/different one to make it work. 'Talk to yourself'.

I've added important details in the way to shift a paradigm and which increased my results in the following method.

1. Acknowledge that this paradigm has been part of your life and the reasons why it was there.

Be grateful it existed in order to detach from it with a positive feeling. It avoids the feeling of denial.
2. Understand this paradigm doesn't benefit you anymore. It is not acceptable to keep it in your life.
3. Think of a positive version of the old paradigm **without using any negation** in your affirmation. Keep positive intentions only. **Think about what it would take to obtain what you want**. If you don't know how, **ask yourself how you succeeded** without trying to find the answer. This will condition your mind to find a solution by itself.
4. Repeat it every day 3 times a day until it becomes your way to think/be/feel.

✎ 1. I accept that my paradigm was ..... It was there because.... Thank you ...
2. I understand that I don't need ... because ... It is not acceptable anymore in my life.
3. From now onwards ... because/ Why ...?
4. Repeat your new habit, affirmation, belief every day to get familiar with it.

Example:
1. I accept that my belief was that I had a poor quality of sleep like my father. Thank you it happened because I now enjoy so much sleeping well.
2. I understand that I don't need this belief anymore because it doesn't benefit me. It is not acceptable anymore in my life.
3. From now onwards, it is so easy to fall asleep, I feel rested and full of energy upon awaking each day. I have healthy habits that explain why I sleep so well or (if you don't know) Why do I sleep so well?

Concentrate on what you want. It's there, you just haven't grabbed it yet, but it's there!

✎ Write down your new tools in your pyramid. 'Switch Button. Spring Cleaning, Paradigm Shift.

VI. STRATEGY- THE LAST PRECIOUS STONE

How to make things work?

A strategy is essential to reach a goal. A 'plan of action' is the keystone that makes all your efforts work on a long term basis.

Wallace Wattles explains in his book *The Science of Getting Rich* that in order to become rich, you need to 'do things a certain way' to get results. [10]

Example: If you are tired and if I give you 2 extra hours, what are you going to do? I would have a restoring nap but you may do something else and not rest. Eventually, you will stay tired whereas I will have recovered and will be more productive at work than you. With the same number of hours we behaved differently which led us to divergent results.

You can understand now that a simple detail in your way of thinking or behaving can make a big difference in your life. Analyse your thoughts and behaviour. The next time a situation repeats itself, do something differently. Here is a way to do things differently.

1. SWITCH THE BUTTON (V)

2. DO SOMETHING NEW AND REPEAT THE PROCESS OVER AND OVER AGAIN

- LEARNING things or acting differently help maintain the connection between the cells of your brain. It encourages neurogenesis (creation of new cells in the brain) and keeps your brain active and strong. The better your brain works, the better it processes information, adopts new habits, and consolidates them. [11]

When new data arrives in the system, it changes the old pattern. And this is exactly what we want.

- REPEAT
You must 'consolidate' the new information or habit you learn in the long term to get results.

The purpose is to become more familiar with the idea or habit. Hence, it has to be easy to access this new information. Repetition is a process that will develop the network used by the brain to access the information recently learnt. The more repetition, the more this information will be easy to access and 'take over' the old beliefs and habits which don't benefit you. It is a case of being willing enough to press the start button and trigger the learning and repetition process.

Why repetition works: science corner

The brain is composed of neurons communicating with each other through live wires called axons. It works like electricity. The neurotransmitters are chemical particles present at the junction where two neurons meet (synapse). They are messengers transferring the information from one axon to another. The axons/wires are protected/insulated thanks to a layer of myelin/insulator (rubber, PVC). Myelin protects the axon from energy/information loss/interferences.

As a result, myelin allows the information to be delivered faster and with better quality. Listen to your favourite music with high quality headphones and do the same with cheap ones. You will now understand the importance of myelin function in the brain.

The higher the demand, the more myelin is produced. When you do push-ups a signal stimulates the cells in your brain that tells your pectoral muscle cells to work. Training makes your body use the same neuropath and type of cells on a higher frequency. The body must produce more myelin in order to cope with the increasing demand (training). The more training, the more myelin is produced.

Eventually, that section of the network used in your brain becomes more insulated, more equipped, and answers better and faster. It has become easier with time and practice to use these pectoral muscles to do push-ups. You become good at it and can perform better. The myelination process needs time to build more myelin, to adjust and be functional the way you want it to be. You must be persistent and patient until it becomes effortless.

Repetition works for everything you do in life (going to the gym, new diet, drinking more water, writing your journal, etc.).

"Practice makes perfect. After a long time of practising, our work will become natural, skillfull, swift and steady."
BRUCE LEE.

Repetition of information makes your brain use the same group of cells. The process is successful once it has become logical and effortless to recall the new information recently learnt and when you think more about it than about the old one. It is similar to developing a new skill or transforming a talent into skill. It refers to the principle of the **Conscious Competence Ladder***. You climb one step at a time as you keep improving your skills in your field of competency.

The first step is when you don't know you have bad habits (or another detrimental emotion or paradigm). The second step is when you know you have bad habits and you know what they are. This awareness allows you to take action, change and build new habits (third step). At last, you reach the fourth step of the ladder and your new habits have become second nature. You don't think about how to do it anymore and you can enjoy the results of your efforts. (12)

3. USE TOOLS TO STAY ON TRACK

Being consistent makes you stick to the exercise, finish your challenge, or keep trying a new routine even if the results are not immediate.

It is a skill you must learn or improve upon to be able to stay on track once you have made a decision.

How to remain consistent
Trying to change everything at once is too much work for your brain which is not used to operating with so many new and different concepts in a short space of time.

A solid step by step procedure with handy tools has more chances to benefit you.
Training with small and new habits on a regular basis will help you build solid foundations in the long term.

1. Make and accept challenges
They keep you active. Motion is energy and motion is action.
A challenge reminds you that there is something you need to do to 'win' or improve your situation. It gives you a feeling of satisfaction or fulfilment when you compete with yourself or your friends or once you have achieved your task. It's entertaining! Be more childlike in your life. Certain things don't have to be so 'serious'!

2. Enjoy teamwork
It maintains the 'pressure' to get things done when you enjoy competing and is a good way to remind you of your goals. A friend can hold you accountable for your capacity to follow the plan you set.

3. Use 'reminders' to encourage repetition
If you are scared of forgetting or usually start to do things and never finish them, three simple solutions exist.

- Set an alarm on your device. You won't have any excuse to forget about the ongoing challenge or exercise.
- Write down your new idea or routine in your diary, put a post-it note on your fridge, and look at it every day.

- Plan tomorrow (chapter 10).

4. Remember to enjoy the process
It's not a punishment to work on being a better version of yourself. It is the 'game of life'! You set goals to bring more satisfaction and happiness in your life and getting results requires action.

Here are some ideas that may remind you and help you enjoy the process when you encounter difficulties.

- Look everyday at your pyramid.
It is your guideline, helps you stay motivated, and makes you think about all the things you've managed to accomplish so far and about what you will achieve soon. It's exciting!

- 'Seduce your elephant'
Petr Ludwig and Adela Schicker explain in their book *End of Procrastination* a Buddhist metaphor of an elephant and a rider. The idea is that you are the rider, the one who thinks and makes the decisions to act. You are the rational brain. [13]

On the other hand, your elephant is the 5 year old child 'in you' who throws a tantrum whenever something goes wrong. It corresponds to your emotions. In order to keep enjoying the process, you need to 'seduce' your elephant, your emotions. Don't ask your elephant to climb the Himalayan Mountain in one day without training. It will run away or kick your butt! Start with the easiest tasks first, one small step at a time. The more small steps are climbed, the bigger the staircase will be climbed, and more things will be accomplished.

- Get excited about this journey and be proud of yourself (only if you are doing something of course).
Feel happy and grateful to be alive because it gives you the opportunity to be who you want to be.

- Use the law of attraction without moderation.
Starting the day in a bad mood isn't usually a good prognostic but if there is some good news you will start smiling again and may have a great day. It is all about energy and good vibes.

The law of attraction works like magnets.
In the book *The Secret* written by Rhonda Byrne and the work of amazing researchers, doctors, philosophers, writers, and many more, the law of attraction is defined by many concepts including the famous 'like attracts like'. [14]

Love attracts love. 'Boredom' attracts boredom. The more happiness and positivity you feel and communicate, the more you will receive in return...the more you enjoy the process, the more positive results you will have...

Enjoy self-development without moderation and it will benefit you. It is a certainty!

✏️ Write down '6. Strategy: learn, repeat, consistency tools' in your pyramid.

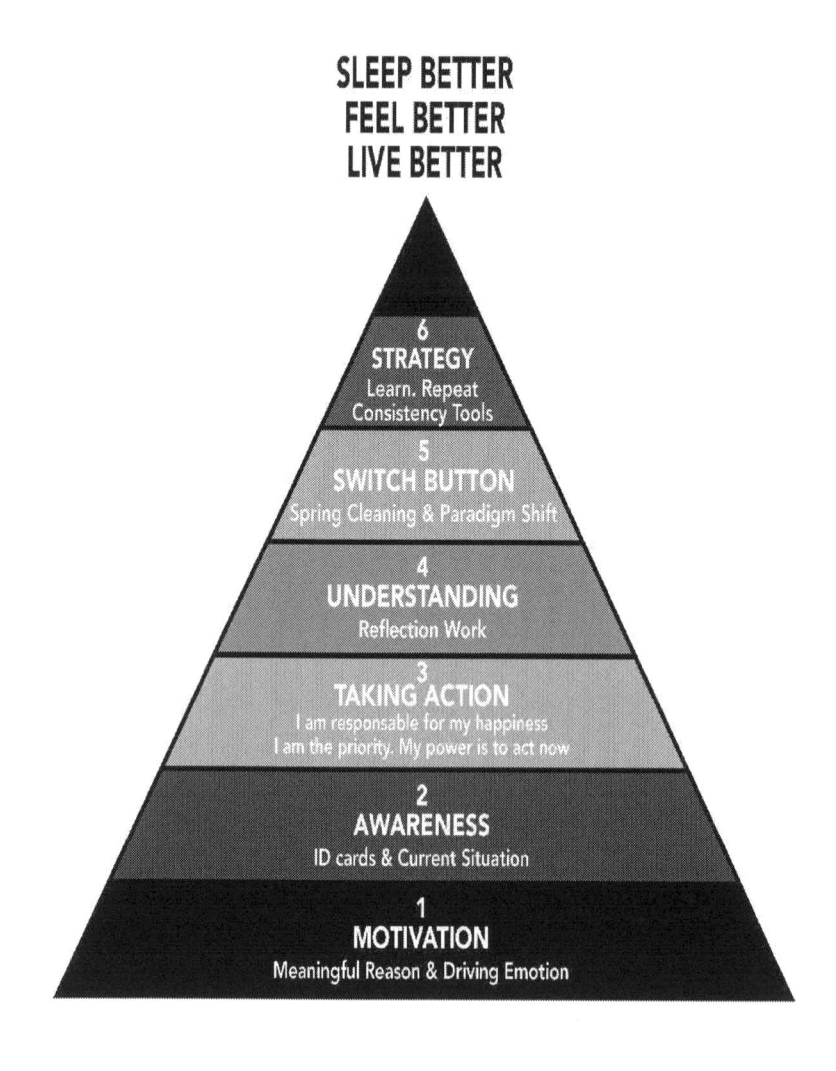

SLEEP BETTER
FEEL BETTER
LIVE BETTER

6 STRATEGY
Learn. Repeat
Consistency Tools

5 SWITCH BUTTON
Spring Cleaning & Paradigm Shift

4 UNDERSTANDING
Reflection Work

3 TAKING ACTION
I am responsable for my happiness
I am the priority. My power is to act now

2 AWARENESS
ID cards & Current Situation

1 MOTIVATION
Meaningful Reason & Driving Emotion

IN A NUTSHELL

• Changing a situation requires more than a simple wish. It is a commitment. There are 6 precious stones you can use during your journey.

• 1. <u>Motivation</u>: find a meaningful reason and a driving emotion to keep you motivated in the process.

• 2. <u>Awareness</u>: assessing your current situation and sleep pattern will help you know where to start and what to do.

• 3. <u>Taking action</u>: You must take responsibility for your life. Time waits for no man. The decision you take to improve your well-being is for you and you alone.

• 4. <u>Understanding</u> yourself is essential to avoid repeating the same mistakes.

• 5. There is a <u>switch button</u> that you have to find in order to obtain results.
- Certain <u>emotions</u> can sometimes be toxic for you and this is why you need to let them go.
- <u>Paradigms</u> can control every part of you and your job is to find them, understand them, and change them into positive ones. Ask yourself what it takes to get to your desired outcome.

• 6. A <u>strategy</u> is necessary to help you consolidate your new habits and keep you on track.

- <u>Learning</u> new things keeps your brain active and repetition is a must for integrating them.
- Challenges, teamwork, and reminders are <u>tools</u> you can use to improve or maintain consistency.
- Always remember to <u>enjoy</u> the process as you go; you are doing this for yourself. Keep your goal and driving emotion in mind and seduce your elephant one small step at a time.
- <u>The Law of Attraction</u> is your best companion. Good actions encourage more good actions and results.
So use it without moderation!

"Those who cannot change their minds cannot change anything."

GEORGE BERNARD SHAW

CHAPTER 4
SELF-ASSESSMENT

Tools you can benefit from in this book
Challenges, exercises, reflection work methods, pyramid, 'in a nutshell' sections, and new concepts or information will help you understand how your brain works and who you are.

Why using tools
Using a tool makes you stay active and increases the chance of obtaining significant results. It is especially useful when you read self-development books as you put what you learn into practice. When correctly used, it allows you to keep track of your progress and remain motivated, therefore consistent.

I. SLEEP PATTERN TOOL - ID CARDS

You need to be aware of the different aspects of your life ('sleep pattern', strengths and weaknesses, dreams and reality, etc.) to identify better what you need and want to improve.
The purpose of these ID cards is to give you an idea of the current quality of your sleep and what you really want.
From this point onwards you will know which direction to take to start improving your situation thanks to the knowledge you will gain from this book. In this book, 'sleep pattern' refers to what corresponds to the main events, habits, thoughts and feelings related to your health and well-being and which can influence the quality of your sleep.

Instructions
- Answer the questions quickly and without over thinking.
- Write down the first thought that comes to your mind. It is usually the best one.
- Choose neither your best days nor the worst ones in order to obtain an average sleep pattern assessment.

1. ID CARD OF YOUR CURRENT SLEEP PATTERN

A. EVERYDAY - ROUTINE
What are your habits? How organised is your life? How stressful is your job or what place does it have in your life?
Do you enjoy your days?

Example: Nothing new happens, work is a bit overwhelming, my days look the same, I'm always stuck in traffic on the way back home for 45 minutes, I go to the liquor store every week, etc.
✎ ...

B. BEDTIME HABITS
How easily do you fall asleep? How busy is your mind when you go to bed? Do you like going to bed? Do you suffer from any ailment that prevents you from sleeping? Do you do something special before you fall asleep?

Example: I have trouble falling asleep because I'm too scared of having nightmares, I usually scroll on Facebook for an hour every day, I cannot afford to go to bed early because I'm too busy,
I have migraines, I love reading when I'm in bed, etc.
✎ ...

C. DURING THE NIGHT
Do you wake up at night? Why do you wake up?

Example: I wake up at 3 am because I'm hungry or I wake up because I need to check how many likes I have on Instagram, etc.
✎ ...

SELF-ASSESSMENT

D. UPON AWAKENING
What do you feel when you wake up? Do you sleep enough?

Example: I usually look forward to the start of a new day or I have no motivation when I wake so I stay in bed for as long as I can. I get enough sleep or I need more sleep.

✎ ...

After answering these questions, summarize the relevant positive and negative key points of the four steps of the day mentioned above. Write down your final current sleep pattern ID on paper.

✎ ...

CURRENT SLEEP PATTERN ID example

Negatives: Boring routine, stressful work, difficulty falling asleep, waking up tired.

Positives: Full night's sleep, happy at breakfast.

CURRENT SLEEP PATTERN ID

Negatives

Positives:

2. ID CARD OF YOUR FUTURE SLEEP PATTERN

A. EVERYDAY - ROUTINE
What kind of good habits would you like to have? How organised would like to be? What would you like to feel about your job? What would make you have good days?

✏️ ...

B. BEDTIME HABITS:
How would you like to fall asleep? What feelings would you like to experience when you go to bed? What would you like to do before you fall asleep?

✏️ ...

C. DURING THE NIGHT:
What would it feel like to sleep without waking up at night? What would you like to dream about?

✏️ ...

D. UPON AWAKENING:
What would you like to feel when you wake up? What would you like to do when you get out of bed every morning?

✏️ ...

FUTURE SLEEP PATTERN ID example

I am organised and can easily disconnect when its bedtime, I read great books everyday, I wake up energised and in good mood. Full night's sleep, breakfast is a happy moment.

FUTURE SLEEP PATTERN ID

.

SELF-ASSESSMENT

✎ *Write down your ideal ID card in your pyramid or stick a post-it the same level as the second precious stone AWARENESS.*

II. CURRENT SITUATION TOOL – ANALYSE

The purpose of the following questions is to make you observe your behaviour, habits or redundant patterns, and enable you to identify more of your strengths and weaknesses. I hope this deeper analysis will make you **understand** your situation better.

How to use it?

- Firstly, be honest with yourself.
- Secondly, use this tool everyday from one to two weeks.
The longer you use it, the more detail you will cover, and the better the results should be.

- Finally, answer quickly as the first thought is often the best one and this is a self-help handbook, not a 5 hour daily exercise.

The questionnaire is made up of three sections.

1. 7, 10 or 14 day challenge questions.
2. Introspection work at the end of section one.
3. Summary of your current situation at the end of the section.

FIRST SECTION: 7, 10 or 14 DAY CHALLENGE

If you remember the details about the past week, you can answer now and keep up with the following days or section 2. Certain questions need to be answered once only (1st question for example).

A. EVERYDAY – ROUTINE

1. Do you work? What is your job? What are your tasks?
How many hours a week do you work?

2. Do you like your job? If you don't have a job, do you want to work and why?

3. Write down three positive and three negative aspects of your job. If you don't have a job what would you like to do and why?

4. Write down any recurrent or new event/task/chore and the time you dedicate to them. How do you feel about it?

5. Did you do all that you wanted or needed to do yesterday? What do you feel about it? What was it?

6. On a scale of 0 to 10, 10 being excellent and 0 being dreadful how was your day yesterday?

7. Write down the driving emotion(s) of yesterday.

Example:
1. Manager in finance in a large company, I lead a team of 11 persons and meet with department heads. 47 hours spent working each week.
2. Don't know if I really like it.
3. <u>Negative</u>: Stressful, underpaid, work too many hours.
   <u>Positive</u>: Responsibilities, possible promotion, overall conscientious and friendly workmates.
4. Stuck in traffic for an hour on the way home every day. I hate it! Had an argument with one employee yesterday but problem solved. The big boss congratulated me on my work. It felt good.
5. Had lunch with an old friend as planned. Great!

SELF-ASSESSMENT

Didn't go to the gym. Damn! Supermarket for 30 minutes. Done.
6. How was my day yesterday: 6/10.
7. This guy at work pissed me off. ANGER. I hate traffic jams. It's a waste of time. FRUSTRATION. Valuable time with my friend. HAPPINESS. It feels good to get a bit of recognition from my boss. SATISFACTION.

✎ ...

B. BEDTIME HABITS

8. Did you want to do something last night? What did you really do?
9. Do you think that you wasted your time yesterday? Were all the things you did necessary? Did they benefit you?
10. Were you feeling good last night? Or were you drained?
11. Write down what you were feeling when you jumped in your bed last night.
12. What were you thinking about?
13. Write down what you were physically feeling once in bed.
14. What time did you go to bed?

Example
8. I wanted to study some German but I watched a TV show instead.
9. I watched a TV show. Not all the things I did yesterday were productive or useful.
10. Really tired. Didn't even eat.
11. I felt guilty because I didn't go to the gym.
12. I was over thinking everything.
13. I was relaxed last night.
14. 11 pm.

✎ ...

C. DURING THE NIGHT

15. Did you wake up during the night? If yes, how many times?
16. Why?
17. What time did you wake up?
18. If you woke up, was it easy to go back to sleep?
19. Do you snore or experience anything unusual when you sleep?

Example
15. Yes, once
16. I don't know.
17. 4 am.
18. Stayed awake for 30 minutes then looked at my phone for
20 minutes then fell asleep
19. No
✎ ...

D. UPON AWAKENING

20. Did you fall asleep easily last night?
21. What time did you wake up this morning?
22. Did you set an alarm? Why?
23. Did you hit the snooze button? How many times?
24. Did you get out of bed immediately?
25. How many hours did you sleep last night?
26. What was your first thought when you woke up today?
27. Were you rested?
28. What emotion did you experience this morning?
29. What were you physically feeling like this morning?

SELF-ASSESSMENT

Example:
20. No, I was overthinking.
21. 6 am.
22. Yes. I was scared of being late for work.
23. Yes, 4 times.
24. No, I waited 30 min (snoozed 4 times).
25. About 6h30.
26. Another mundane day.
27. I was a bit tired.
28. I wasn't excited to start the day.
29. I needed to stretch.
✎ ...

SECOND SECTION: INTROSPECTION WORK

These questions are related to the first sections. They encourage you to understand your responsibilities, to find a solution, or see the situation from another point of view.

Questions 1, 2, and 3 (section one) refer to your career or job's expectations.

Introspection work: **Weigh the pros and cons of your current situation and find a solution if you don't feel satisfied and fulfilled.**

Feeling disturbed when it comes to important aspects of your life can lead to unhappiness or to over think when it's bedtime. Being satisfied and fulfilled often involves 'you' identifying and choosing what is good for you 'regardless' of what other people think (principles, family, friends or people's opinion, religion, culture, etc.). These different elements have varying degrees of importance for different people but the key point is to understand that they have a significant impact on the human brain. They condition the way you think, the way you feel and behave.

55

Eventually, your life tends to become what others make it and not what you want to make it.

Some of the beliefs or habits you have developed over the years because of your environment and experiences can lead to self-sabotage of your dreams and goals.

Bear in mind, as well, that these same beliefs or habits can seem 'illogical or unthinkable' to others.

Maintaining a certain balance in every aspect of your life would help you feel satisfied and fulfilled (family, friends, principles, etc. shouldn't take too much importance in your decision making).

For example, you would like to be a manager but you grew up thinking you weren't clever enough because your family has told you so. This belief prevents you from becoming a manager, which may seem 'illogical or unthinkable' to your friends who think you are capable.

The truth is that nobody else but you lives your life. You are who you want to be and not who someone else wants you to be.

Do what you want because this is your wish and nobody is responsible for your happiness except you.

You are the **priority** (taking action – priority).

a. What do you want?
b. Have you done something to change your situation? Why?
c. What could you do to get what you want?

Example:
a. I want to work somewhere else.
b. I haven't done anything about it because I'm too busy with my children.
c. I could rearrange my schedule to take the time to write a CV.

🖉 ...

Question 4 (section one) refers to your attitude (emotion + belief + behaviour) regarding repetitive situations or last minute events.

Introspection work: Analyse your attitude regarding the different aspects of your life you referred to in section one and find a solution.

Any repetitive and annoying event can be sorted out. There is always a way if you are 'willing' enough to change the situation.

d. What are the repetitive or unexpected events that you have experienced during the last 7, 10, or 24 days?
e. Write down your overall attitude.
f. What could you do to make it different if it disturbs you? What different attitude could you have?

Example
d. Traffic jams.
e. Attitude: getting angry but not changing anything.
f. He could avoid rush hour by changing his working hours if possible because he's the manager, or listen to German courses when he's stuck in traffic.

✎ ...

Question 5 (section one) what would you have loved to do? Did you do it?

Introspection work: Observe your ability to listen to yourself, to your needs and find a solution.

Firstly, doing something you love every day is a way to treat yourself ... 'with love'. It maintains a balance between the 'agreeable' and 'less agreeable' tasks of the day.
Secondly, this moment recharges 'your batteries' by giving the energy boost you need to accomplish your daily tasks especially when you suffer from sleep deprivation.

Give yourself 30 minutes a day (or more if possible) to do what you enjoy doing.

**g. Do you do something you enjoy doing everyday? Why?
If the answer is no, what could you do?**

Example:
g. No because I don't have enough time.
I could play the guitar or study some German courses.
🖉 ...

Question 5 + Do you do everything which you intended to do every day?)

Introspection work: Observe how productive your schedule allows you to be. Find a way to improve your schedule if you need to.

Achieving all your tasks every day brings you satisfaction, relief, and avoids generating useless stress that can sometimes be overwhelming when you go to bed.
Track how much you procrastinate or waste time doing unnecessary things and rethink your schedule.

**h. Do you usually do what needs to be done? Why?
i. How could you do it differently?**

Example:
h. I often postpone what needs to be done because I don't like doing certain tasks.
i. I could discipline myself to do what I don't like doing in order to avoid keeping this useless 'pressure' in my mind all day long.
🖉 ...

Questions 6 and 7 refers to your general well-being.

Introspection work: Assess how happy you are and remember what makes you feel good.

SELF-ASSESSMENT

Rating your day gives you an overall idea of how happy you are, on average. Most days should score more than 7 out 10.
Over thinking, overwhelming negative emotions, or not enough time out can lead to low scores and sleep problems.

j. Write down the average of the score you wrote during the last 7, 10, or 14 days. Is it equal to or above 7 out of 10?
k. What could bring 'sunshine' to your days and improve this score?

Example:
j. 6.5/10
k. I could spend more time with my friends and do more what I enjoy (painting, playing music, etc.).
✎ ...

l. Do you feel recurrent negative and strong emotions during the day?
m. How could you work on this kind of emotion?

Introspection work: pointing at toxic elements, situations, or people in your life you need to step away from.

Whereas negatives pull you down in all aspects of your life, positive emotions make you feel good. Sounds logical? A happy state of mind can make you feel capable of achieving anything and this is why you must focus on the people and things that make you feel good.

> 'I don't have time to worry about who doesn't like me.
> I'm too busy loving the people who love me.'
> UNKNOWN

Example:
l. Recurrent negative emotions: frustration and anger because of daily traffic jam.

Lack of confidence due to being overweight.
m. New plan to handle traffic better (podcast, audio books, music).
Reiki treatment to help balance your emotions, or any other active option such as practising a physical activity.

✎ ...

Questions 8, 9, 10, and 20 refer to your time and energy.

Introspection work: Assess the way you use your time, the relevance of your actions and their energy expenditure.

Observing if you manage to follow your plans shows how good you are at using your time properly.
Observing your productivity and the energy cost of your actions/tasks enables you to prioritise, eventually saving some energy.

n. Do you usually follow your plans? Why? How much does your environment interfere with your life? How could you do it differently?

Example:
n. No. I multitask and don't always finish what I have to do. Taking care of my children requires a lot of effort.
I should learn to concentrate on one thing at a time. I could make my children busy with musical or artistic activities.

✎ ...

o. Do you prioritize your tasks? Write down the consequences in your life of not prioritizing. If no, how could you do better?

Example:
o. I don't always prioritize. I leave big chores to deal with until the end of the day when I'm too tired to deal with them. Eventually, I spend my day off dealing with them.

SELF-ASSESSMENT

I could start with the most energy demanding task in the morning and do a bit each day.

✎ ...

You have a certain amount of energy available to use every day. The less you have to think, the more energy you save.
Starting with the 'biggest' task or the one you hate the most increases your self-discipline which is an essential skill that makes you accomplish your tasks/goals. On the other hand, doing it at the end of the day may be harder because you have less energy. Logical, isn't it?

Settings plans and prioritizing will help you get more things done and prevent this frustration and dissatisfaction of non-productivity.

p. Are all the things you usually do useful?

Certain things don't need to be done in one day or don't need to be done at all. Being aware of these things and reorganising your time with actions that benefit you will improve your productivity and save you some energy.

Example: It is difficult to work full time, go to the supermarket, do your laundry, clean the house, go to the gym, take care of your children and give yourself some valuable time all in one day. Instead, delegate or set up a weekly task plan.

✎ ...

q. Do you have some time or energy left at the end of the day? If no, how can you make it different? What would you do if you had more time and energy everyday?

Analyse your activities and find, if possible, anytime during the day that could be used differently.
There is a difference between feeling drained and experiencing a good fatigue. The first option requires a change of plan which

can start with small changes if your life is hectic (strategy -seduce your elephant).

Examples
q. I have 30 minutes of 'free' time everyday but I'm exhausted.
I could go to bed earlier instead of watching TV shows everyday. It may help me feel better.

My children drain all the energy out of me. I never rest. I must set limits. I could find a way to keep them busy with a physical activity for instance. I could enjoy my time when I'm alone.

✎ ...

Questions 11, 12, 13 refer to your general mindset

Introspection work: observe if there is good harmony between your emotions, your thoughts and your health.

The way you think and feel impacts on your health and vice versa. Superfluous wishes, negative thoughts and emotions can prevent you from feeling good, this is why you need to work on them (spring cleaning, paradigm shift, or other methods).

Your health tells you a lot about your life.
Emotions are trapped in a certain form, in a certain way, at a certain place and time in your body.
Dis-ease is expressed when there is something you are not comfortable with and your job is to find a solution to this discomfort. Sleep disorders can cause physical and emotional pain in the long run and vice versa.

r. Write down some of the repetitive thoughts and emotions you may experience every day.
s. Write down the positive version if they are negative.

SELF-ASSESSMENT

t. Do you feel fit and healthy? What do you feel? Does what you physically feel influence your emotions and decisions and vice versa? What would you like to feel and what could you do to reach this goal?

Example:
r. I regularly think about my job and what I don't like about it.
s. I'm happy with my new schedule or I'm happy I have a new job or I'm happy I work in a different team...
t. No. I feel tired too often. It makes me procrastinate a lot.
I would like to have more energy and strength. I could sleep more/participate in a sport/change my diet/have a break...
✎ ...

Questions 14, 21, 25 refer to your habits

Irregular 'time habits' force your body to work harder to readjust and cope with the energy demand of the day.
Eventually, it leads to chronic fatigue. Maintaining a balanced rhythm helps your internal body clock work properly, therefore allowing you to accomplish your tasks smoothly and 'effortlessly'.

u. Do I have a bedtime routine?
v. What could you do to be more consistent in your habits?

Example:
u. No
v. I could go to bed at the same time every night and earlier than 11 pm.
✎ ...

Questions 15 to 18, 27, and 29 refer to your 'night habits'.

Introspective work: highlights if there is a reason why you wake up and how you deal with it.

Repetitive wakes can disturb your sleep cycles which become incomplete and inefficient. Eventually, it may have some repercussions on your health.

There is a bunch of possible reasons you are waking up at night; full bladder, a few alcoholic drinks, heavy dinner, sleep apnoea, worries, restless leg syndrome, etc. Waking up at the same time may refer to unhealed emotions linked to the function of an organ. I suggest you read about Chinese Medicine Clocks. You can find many of these clocks online. If waking up doesn't happen repetitively, you shouldn't check the time because it may condition your mind (unconsciously) to feel the need to wake up again at the same time. Besides, the light of your phone (if it's in your room) will keep you awake longer.

Always refer to your doctor in case of doubt or unusual signs.

w. Do you wake up at night and why?
x. How do you handle your wake-ups?
y. Does it affect your physical feelings in the morning or for the rest of the day?
z. What could you do to make it better?

Example:
w. Yes but I don't know why.
x. I stare at my phone for 20 minutes at least.
y. Yes. I feel a bit tired upon wakening.
z. I could avoid looking at my phone and get regular bedtime hours.

✎ ...

Question 19 refer to possible medical issues

Introspection work: Recognize when you should ask for help or support.

Any abnormal symptom requires more attention. Snoring and apnoea may cause oxygen deprivation to the brain and need to be assessed. You may ask your partner if you snore or stop breathing during your sleep.
Refer to a doctor for advice or further investigations.
Restless leg syndrome might be caused by a hormonal disorder or something else and needs a medical opinion.

🖉 ...

Questions 22 to 28 refer to your morning state of mind.

Introspection work: assess the harmony between your body, mind and emotions.

Our thoughts and feelings can influence our actions. 'The way' you wake up is a good indication on your internal body clock regulation, your average state of mind, and the possible foremost emotions in your life.

There are several reasons why people set morning alarms.
Your job is to analyse if you really need them.

Firstly, you may not need to set an alarm as you wake up anyway but it is 'just in case' to ensure you'll be on time for work or an appointment.
Secondly, it is a simple weekly habit that conditions your life. You could turn it off during the weekend to learn to relax (?).
Last but not least, it is a necessity in order to wake up. This can reveal a general lack of motivation or a certain imbalance in your habits such as irregular bedtimes leading to the need to sleep

more. Your job is to understand why you struggle to wake up and to find a meaningful reason to be happy to wake up every day.

This possible lack of motivation is confirmed with the use of the 'snooze button'. A smart and 'terrible' invention at the same time, it pushes people to act urgently, '5 more minutes, 5 more minutes, until s***! I'm late'. It creates a loop of useless stress and wastes your time and energy. You might think it 'allows you' to sleep longer but it can break your sleep cycle instead. It eventually reduces the quality of your sleep. To sum it up, using a snooze button is no better than procrastinating.

Although everyone is unique, it is a good idea to observe the habits of the ones around you who sleep well. They might not need to set an alarm every day because their internal body clock is very well regulated and/or because they enjoy their life.

a. What do you feel and think about when you hear the alarm upon awakening?
b. Is a snooze button necessary?
c. Do your morning emotions/feelings control your actions/behaviour?
d. Are your habits encouraging a well-balanced life?
e. What positive impact can your decisions have on your life?

Example:
a. I feel **tired** upon awakening and I'm **scared** of not waking up if I don't use an alarm.
b. I feel like snoozing makes me sleep longer but I'm still tired.
c. I'm **tired** which forces me to drink 5 coffees a day to stay awake at work. My **job** isn't an **incentive** to get me out of bed.
d. My bedtime habits: I go to bed too late and at irregular times which means that I don't sleep enough.
e. I must go to bed earlier to feel more rested.

I have to find another job that gives me reasons to wake up in a good mood.

✎ ...

SITUATION TABLE

	Does it benefit you?	How long since it started?	What do you feel about it?	Did you do something to try 'fixing' it	Are you 'willing' to change it?	Opposite version of the negatives
Repetitive Thoughts						
Repetitive Emotions						
Repetitive Habits						
Repetitive Behaviour						
Weaknesses						

THIRD SECTION: RESUME OF YOUR CURRENT SITUATION.

This section summarizes the habits, beliefs, thoughts and feelings that may be toxic for your well-being.

Consider asking a trustworthy person to hold you accountable for your reflection work and the decisions you may make after spending time reflecting on this last section. It can bring more objectivity to your analysis because we often tend to deny things, and it may increase your consistency (strategy-teamwork).

✎ *Summarize your answers in the following 'situation table'.*

🖊 Highlight the keywords in sections one and two. Write them down on this table. They are the elements you need to take into account to improve your situation.
🖊 Stick this table to your pyramid.
🖊 What would it take to turn your 'demons' into positive outcomes? (look at your pyramid)
🖊 Write down your strengths and positive habits/ thoughts/ behaviour /emotions in your pyramid. They are tools you can use to help you in your self-development journey.

The following chapters (5 to the end) will give you more support and advice to help you change your thoughts, emotions, habits, behaviour, and eventually, make you sleep, feel, and live better.

Any abnormal symptom requires specific attention. If you have or may have a condition, you should seek medical advice. You must understand this statement and take the necessary actions if needed.

IN A NUTSHELL

- A tool is an essential key instrument meant to maintain your level of consistency. It tracks your progress, encourages action, and therefore increases the chance of having better results.

- The tools presented here are; the ID cards of your sleep pattern, the introspection work you accomplish through the self-assessment questionnaire, and the pyramid you draw.

- ID cards summarise your current and desired sleep pattern.

- Your sleep pattern corresponds to your behaviour, habits, daily events, feelings, and thoughts that can influence the quality of your sleep. It relies on what happens in your 24/7 routine and how you feel about it.

- A self-assessment is essential to understand oneself. You can cover one to two weeks of your life's habits and mindset with the questionnaire offered in this chapter. It outlines the main weaknesses you need to work on to improve your well-being.

- The introspection work covers many aspects of your life
    - The pros and cons of your job-related situation
    - Your overall attitude regarding some of the events in your life
    - Your self-love and self-esteem level
    - Your organisation skills
    - Your degree of happiness
    - How you deal with your negatives
    - Your relationship with time and energy
    - Your emotional balance and your self-care level
    - What controls you

- This chapter gives you a taste of how to acknowledge your strengths and weaknesses and gives you the opportunity to turn the negatives into positives.

- Draw your pyramid with the key elements you obtained from the chapter 3 and 4. You have now a starting point and a clearer direction to follow. Start climbing the ladder!

"We are what we repeatedly do.
Excellence then, is not an act, but a habit".
ARISTOTLE.

CHAPTER 5
BASICS AND HABITS

I. HOLISTIC APPROACH OF YOUR BODY

Having a good night's sleep maintains a good balance in all aspects of your life. As an osteopath, I naturally praise the holistic approach we should have on our body. So, take a minute and imagine you accidentally stuck chewing gum to your jumper. As you try to remove it, the fibres go with it because it is sticky. Sounds logical? Our body functions the same way. Everything is interconnected [1]; your brain, your body, and what makes you unique; your mind and spirit. If one is unbalanced, the others will try to create an 'acceptable' balance in the body to maintain its good homeostasis and survival, at least for a certain time.

When an area of the body is out of balance, it has to compensate somewhere else to be able to preserve its main functions. Eventually, imbalance creates imbalance. When the compensations are too numerous to handle or use too much energy, tensions, dis-ease and-or pain appear.

For example, if you hurt your left shoulder, the right shoulder may have to work more to compensate for the weakness in the affected limb. Tension may occur in your 'good' shoulder, then in your neck, and if certain physical or emotional events happen, migraines or something else may subsequently appear. You can apply this principle to the rest of the body. If you drink too much alcohol, your liver will work harder therefore you may feel more 'tired' than you should and so on.

Your job is to eliminate or reduce what can create imbalances in your life.

Self-help methods and information presented in this book can support you in this task but always bear in mind that you must seek professional advice regarding potential health conditions.

Your negative thoughts, feelings and beliefs lead to negative behaviours, actions and habits and vice versa. A poor quality of sleep creates imbalances in your body and vice versa.

Some healthy habits and advice are discussed below. They are 'easy' to put into action and tend to reduce any unnecessary tension in your body.

Remember that you need to 'seduce your elephant' (emotions) with small and easy changes to remain motivated and consistent in your actions (chapter 3- enjoy the process).

II. ATMOSPHERE AND SLEEP

Treating yourself with love and esteem encourages positive results. The atmosphere you create in your house, in your bedroom are very much related to your feelings. Therefore, creating nice living conditions will help you sleep and feel better. An uncluttered home and life is essential and contribute to maintaining a healthy lifestyle. However, they are too often underestimated. Many people who suffer from sleep disorders live in untidy houses and have unhealthy habits.

YOUR SLEEPING AREA

1. TV in your bedroom

You should keep your TV away from your bedroom. It tends to keep you awake longer because of its artificial light. Electronic devices distract us from the real world and the present moment.

Its addictive side takes over the desire we have to communicate with our partner/relatives and may even impact on our sexual life. Keep your bedroom for its only purpose, to sleep, rest, or make babies...if you wish.

2. Phone in your bedroom
Phones emit radio frequencies and are a source of distraction while you sleep (notifications or messages from your friends/relatives). Get into the habit of turning on the flight mode button to concentrate more on your sleep. Imagine what you could do without a phone in your room. How would you use your time and how it would feel? For example, you could read a book which is great for your brain and less harsh for your eyes and you could enjoy the silence.

✎ Write down on paper every time you look at your phone/tablet for no specific reason (important appointment), and count the time spent on it, every day, and for 7 days. At the end of this week ask yourself how you could use the time you wasted. Set the challenge to keep your phone away from your bedroom for 7 days then write down how you feel and all the things you do instead.

3. Home de-cluttering
Sleeping in an organized and clean room is more agreeable than 'meeting' smelly socks on your way to bed. It is a psychological factor that promotes a better sleep onset

Geek info: 30 000 to 40 000 skin cells fall off your body every hour, which means that you lose about 320 000 skin cells per night in your bed and... on your pillow. (2) Changing bed sheets at least once every two weeks and pillow cases every week will avoid a build-up of food for arachnids in your bed. These little night companions are very keen to eat you and can cause allergies, asthma, infections, etc.!

4. Temperature in the bedroom
If you remember, your body needs to cool down to allow an easier sleep onset (chapter two).

Too warm isn't good as it 'prevents' your lungs from working properly and too cold isn't comfortable for obvious reasons. The ideal temperature is between 16 to 19 degrees Celsius (60 to 67 degrees Fahrenheit). [3]

Adjusting the temperature of your room helps your body save energy and promote an easier sleep onset.

'SLEEPING GEAR'

Your mattress is a key element in the quality of your sleep. It shouldn't be too soft as it doesn't provide good support for your back nor too hard as it isn't comfortable.

Fact: If you hesitate between buying the latest Nintendo or a good mattress, remember that you sleep about one-third of your life whereas a new Nintendo version (or other brand) will probably be released in less than a year!

> 'I have the most expensive mattress from New Zealand, 2000 dollars, the best buy in ten years marriage'.
> MARISOL, A FRIEND OF MINE

This made me laugh a lot but her true testimony explains how important certain 'details' can be.

Your pillow should be at the height that keeps your head and your spine aligned on the same horizontal plan. It prevents you away from neck pain and tension. If you already suffer from a sore neck, I highly suggest you get the right pillow to reduce your pain and- or prevent further complications.

TRY FENG SHUI TO BOOST YOUR SERENITY.

General information.

Feng Shui means Wind Water and is a very ancient (4000 BCE) pseudoscience that was been developed in China. [4]

It is the Art of organising your living space in a way that will make you feel good, relaxed, and energized. Different principles apply for each room in a house and are related to the kind of frequency you want to maintain. A bedroom is 'about' serenity whereas a working space requires more stimulating energies.

The purpose of Feng Shui is to arrange the chi=energy in order to create a balance between the energies yin (feminine passive) and Yan (masculine active) in your living space. The main benefit is to bring some positive energies into your life. (5)

For the most sceptical minds, ask yourself this question:
Do you sleep better after a bad day or a great day?
Although there is a lot to say about the topic, I will only discuss a few Feng Shui tips which I feel are essential to consider. Your living space is often the image of what is happening in your life; your thoughts, feelings and relationships. When you feel stuck or cannot make a decision, think about what your working space, your home or your bedroom look like. Everything holds energy. Solids, liquids, and gas are made of molecules that move. (6)

Moving your furniture or changing their appearance modifies the frequencies emitted in your environment. It creates an energy shift and prevents the stagnation of old energies which are detrimental to your well-being. (7)

In Feng Shui, energy shifts bring good vibes therefore making you feel better and satisfied instantly. It is visual and emotional.

Example: Refer to the nice feeling you have every time you finish your housework. You're happy, satisfied, and with a smile on your face you probably say 'Done!'

Banish mirrors from your bedroom and especially the ones facing the bed. They can create discomfort for you or your partner. The reflection effect of the mirror, laptop or TV in the room creates a strange sensation that a 'third party' is in the bedroom. If you can't remove it, add a curtain or something neutral to cover it.

Windows behind the bed.
Visible windows behind the bed bring too much yin chi in the room. They can be a source of energy disturbance and may enhance nightmares. Simply close the curtains when you want to sleep. (5)

Colours
Too much yang chi in your bedroom stimulates the mind which may keep you awake longer. The yang chi colours such as red, yellow and orange, are ideal for working areas. (8) Instead bring more yin chi by choosing gentle and neutral colours to obtain a safe, cosy and peaceful atmosphere. The yin chi colours are brown, cream, gentle purple, blue or green. They are relaxing and grounding.

Remove pictures of people in your room.
Too much decoration gives the feeling of a busy room. It feels like having a crowd watching you sleep (you don't live with Harry Potter at Hogwarts School). (5)

Light keeps you awake (see circadian rhythm further in this chapter). Sleep in the dark or use a very soft and relaxing light at the side of your bed. A spotlight is more direct and harsh in the room. Himalayan Salt Lamps have amazing effects on people. They have become popular over the last few years as they soothe the atmosphere with their pretty and calming pink glow colours.

III. MAGNETIC FIELDS

While some people are adamant that sleeping with the head pointing 'north' isn't a good thing (in India for instance), others claim that this is of no importance.

Some experiments have proved that our brain may be unconsciously capable of sensing the Earth's magnetic field. Studies show the impact of this kind of strength on the brain. Researchers have recorded a change in the brainwave patterns while applying a magnetic field towards the ground on a person facing 'north'. We need more studies on the topic but the results found could help us understand why some people sleep better while facing a certain direction. [9]

Try to sleep in different directions if you have headaches or bad dreams and choose what is best for you. It is like a sixth sense!

IV. LISTEN TO YOUR BODY

Go to bed when you are tired.
Some days are more energy demanding than others. Don't prevent your body from resting longer if you need it. Staying awake instead of going to bed when you're tired will only cause more fatigue and may cause daytime sleepiness at work or on the road. There is no right or wrong time, no exact amount of hours to sleep but whatever makes you feel good. Everybody is unique and has their own needs.

V. SHOWER AND SLEEP

A morning shower is a good way to boost your day. It wakes you up and makes you feel warm or fresh. Although, an evening shower has great effects on your sleep as well. A warm bath full of bubbles or a long warm shower allow your body to relax, therefore it is easier to fall asleep. [10] Not only does an evening shower clean you physically and get rid of the sweat from your body, it also cleans you on an emotional level. It creates this sensation of relief that all the tension is over, or this kind of pleasure you feel when you jump into your fluffy bed!

A good exercise is to visualize the water washing away all the negative thoughts as it pours down your skin.

Imagine all the stress and anxiety being washed away.

Remember to shower one to two hours before bedtime as your body needs to cool off for a better sleep onset. You should start feeling 'a bit chilly' when its bed time. Listen to your body!

VI. SPORT AND SLEEP

You have to love sport! It has to be your best friend, as much as your dog could be (if you have one). A regular physical activity benefits your life. But do you know why? And do you do any sport at all?

...

Practising a physical activity on a regular basis regulates your entire system. It 'helps you maintain your circadian rhythm'. [11]
It trains you to breathe better by using your diaphragm and regulates your blood pressure. It warms up your muscles, therefore reducing tension in the body. A regular sport session makes you feel good as it releases happiness hormones called 'endorphins'. These are responsible for this 'high' feeling you experience after a 30 minute jog for example. [12]

Certain sports are great for calming you down such as a gentle yoga session or some Tai chi because they teach you how to regulate your energy and control your breathing.
Although all sports are a source of well-being. Tennis teaches you to 'play with energies'. You transfer energy to the other player through the ball with more or less intensity. Both players have to adjust their strength and intention while sending back the ball. It's a game of 'energy'. Running, cycling, and swimming are excellent for your endurance and cardio-pulmonary functions. Gymnastics or rock climbing will emphasize more on your strength and technique but are excellent for your endurance as well.
Consider swimming if you suffer from joint injuries as it allows you to work out without the weight of your own body operating against your moves (gravity).

It is essential to build up our activity. For example, if you have never run before, start with short walks then longer ones. Eventually add short running sessions of 10 minutes for example, until you are capable of running 30 to 40 minutes or more at once. Take your time to let your body adjust to the new energy demand.

If you're not familiar with physical exercise, ask a sport coach or other professional to help you do it correctly.

When to practise your activity is up to you. (13) It can be part of your morning routine or whenever you dedicate time to yourself.

Example: I prefer running at the end of the day as it releases the tension of the day and gives me the satisfaction of task achievement. Running in the morning makes me feel 'too relaxed' or sleepy and I may need 2 hours rest and a double shot of caffeine to stimulate my brain to return to an active state!
So, put on your nicest sport outfit and go grab some endorphins!

VII. 'PROTECT' YOUR BRAIN

You probably suffer from sleep disorders but have never visited a doctor to eliminate a possible medical condition related to your brain function. However this medical check may help you recover faster or improve your health.

You cannot do anything without a functional brain. It supports your nervous system which controls the vital functions of your body. It allows you to move your little toe as well as creating a Microsoft Empire, if you'd like to.

Geek info: your brain weights about 1,5kg and 77-78% of it is water. On top of this, you dehydrate as you age which means that it gets smaller with old age. (14) So you'd better take care it!

How to protect it only requires healthy habits and a certain amount of common sense. Although, studies show how much people underestimate the importance of taking care of it. Our brain is protected by the skull, the meninges, liquids and other soft tissues. It is 'floating' in the skull. It is vulnerable and a single shock or repetitive trauma can cause injuries, brain diseases, and even death.

The most common injuries are called concussions.
A concussion mostly occurs after a head trauma and temporarily prevents your brain from functioning at optimum capacity. Head traumas generally occur following accidents or intense practice while undertaking certain physical activities such as rugby, boxing, football, skiing, horse riding or cycling. These traumas can happen in your everyday life as well.

The symptoms you may present after an injury due to intense migraines, dizziness, nausea and vomiting, loss of consciousness, confusion, drowsiness and other unusual symptoms such as convulsions or seizures. [15]

Car accidents are well-known for causing **whiplash.** During this kind of trauma, your brain hits the skull and eventually bruises (because your brain is a muscle).
The symptoms you may present with are too numerous to mention but the main ones are migraines, neck pain, stiffness of your entire body, trouble sleeping and focusing, minor to extreme fatigue, blurred vision, confusion, etc.

Head injuries and sleep

As we just mentioned when your brain is injured, it cannot function to its best potential. A recent or old head trauma can cause symptoms which affect your sleep pattern. Any intensity of head trauma is enough to disturb the brain's functions and the blow doesn't have to be strong to cause injuries.

A United States Study undertaken by the department of Neurology in The Northshore University Health System, shows that between 30% and 70% of the people who had sustained head injuries were presenting with sleep disorders and/or developed symptoms such as pain or anxiety that impacted on the quality of their sleep. [16]

Several studies amongst a population of children and adults showed a persistence in the symptoms up to two years after the head trauma occurred.

If you suffer from a sleep disorder, ask yourself if you have any other symptoms related to concussion and whiplash. Have you ever had any head trauma?

Consequences of head traumas on your health

Head traumas may cause irreversible health conditions ranging from light to severe intensity; from a simple difficulty remembering new things/names, being uncoordinated in your movements for a few days to years, or to an internal bleeding that can threaten your life.

1. The Basics but good habits checklist

1. Wearing a helmet considerably decreases any potential serious head trauma. In 2018 in the United Sates, 857 cyclists died on the road. It represents 2.1 % of fatalities and 'the highest number since 1990'. Studies found that the use of helmets reduces the odds of head injuries by 50% (December 2018). Not less than 83% of deaths involved people NOT wearing a helmet. [17] Have you always worn a helmet when you should have? I have suffered from concussion and whiplash in my life and consider myself lucky that I have only suffered from slight memory loss and trouble learning or focusing on my studies for a few years.

2. Seek medical advice if you have just suffered a head trauma and have some unusual symptoms.
3. Regular health check-ups are a good way to reduce the risk of disease when you practise a sport that exposes you to high risks of head traumas.
4. Resting.
You need to slow down or completely stop your physical activity for a few days or weeks. Accumulating traumas creates tension in your body that is detrimental to your health in the long term and can reduce your performance. Your body needs time to recover properly. Sport keeps you fit and healthy. On the other hand, it tires your body if the activity is not balanced with breaks.

2. The good diet for your brain.

There is a connection between your brain and what you eat.
The gut is the second brain of our body.

Our Nervous System is organised in two parts, Central and Peripheral which communicate with each other. [18]
The Central Nervous System (CNS) is made up of the brain and the spinal cord. It's a control centre that deals with sensory and visceral information.

The Peripheral Nervous System (PNS) is composed of 12 Cranial nerves and 31 Spinal nerves. It comprises the Somatic System (body) and the Autonomic System.
The Autonomic system corresponds to the Sympathetic nerves, and Parasympathetic nerves (PS) that are involved in the digestive process (our gut). It tells us when to rest and digest.

In simple terms, the second brain (our gut) communicates with the first brain (CNS) and if one function is disturbed the other may follow. Everything is interconnected.

Sleep and appetite

The regulation of these elements works in two ways.

Sleep balances the level of hormones that regulate the appetite: ghrelin and leptin. When you suffer from sleep deprivation, the level of leptin drops and ghrelin increases. This imbalance stimulates the appetite and can result in cravings which, if satisfied, can lead to weight gain. [19]

On the other hand, eating at regular times and providing your brain with good nutrients helps maintain a good flow of chemicals which are essential to regulate your body and its functions (sleep, digestive process, breathing, etc.).

On a scale of 1 to 10, 1 being poor and 10 being excellent,
- How good is the quality of your sleep?
- How good are your food habits? (eating at regular times, type of diet).
- Score the balance between the quality of your sleep and your food habits.

Do you experience some cravings from time to time? How often? Why do you feel the need to eat? What emotion do you experience before, during and after your secret snack?
(Refer to chapter 3; spring cleaning, paradigm shift).

A. THE BRAIN ENEMIES AND BAD HABITS

1) Coffee and other caffeinated products

Coffee has a psychoactive effect on the human brain and is one of the most widely consumed drugs in the world. It contains a molecule called caffeine and so do other sources of food and drinks such as certain chocolate, sodas, energy drinks, tea, guarana and even decaffeinated pills! [20]

Caffeine (coffee, tea, etc.) has many effects on the body and here are the main ones. It gives you a morning boost, stimulates your system and is a good excuse to socialize with people.

Although, if the consumption of caffeine is non-regulated or consumed to an extreme it can cause heart palpitations, anxiety, irritability, and other negative effects. [21]

Your brain is a place of chemical reactions regulated by complex systems involving all sorts of chemicals (e.g.: hormones, neurotransmitters).

How does caffeine prevent you from sleeping?
Your body needs to create energy to enable you to move and live normally. To create energy, your body breaks down a molecule called ATP which is created by tiny factories called mitochondria. After breaking down this molecule, the body releases A, T and P. The A is called Adenosine. This Adenosine molecule has to find an empty Adenosine receptor to create a complex. This triggers a chemical reaction that inhibits the activity of the neurons responsible for keeping you awake. Adenosine makes you feel sleepy.

Late afternoon coffees
Caffeine can fix onto the same receptor as the adenosine. It creates the complex caffeine - Adenosine Receptor which prevents the adenosine molecule from finding empty adenosine receptors. This complex triggers the opposite reaction by inhibiting that which inhibits the neurons activity. Therefore, it stimulates the neurons that keep you awake.

How long the caffeine affects your body is a subjective question as it depends on the type of drink and your habits. [22] The more coffee you drink the less sensitive you are to the effects of caffeine. It works like an 'addiction'. Most researchers reveal that caffeine takes between 10 and 20 minutes to take effect on the body and about 40 to 45 minutes to reach its peak of effect. [23]

When should we drink our last cup of coffee?
The American Academy of Sleep Medicine discovered that it takes for a 10 mg consumption, about 5 hours for the body to get rid of half of the substance (effect of the caffeine on the system). [23-24]

These results depend on many factors of course but it gives you an overall idea of when you should drink your last coffee. A double espresso in Europe is about 125mg of caffeine! If you are not a big coffee drinker, don't drink an espresso after 5 pm! The Academy advises you to have your last shot of coffee at least 6 hours before bedtime.

Stopping your coffee habits can make the receptors that receive the caffeine in your brain disappear. A few days or weeks are enough to notice a higher sensitivity to smaller doses and reduce the presence of the chemical in your system.

2) Other drugs that don't benefit your brain

Cocaine, heroin, nicotine, opium, and excess alcohol are well-known for their toxic effect on health. They increase the level of dopamine in your system, a brain chemical that regulates essential functions of the body. When its flow is unbalanced, moderate to severe health conditions can occur. A significant low level of dopamine is associated with Parkinson's disease. An excess of dopamine is found with Schizophrenia. [25]

Cigarettes contain nicotine which is a brain stimulant. Smoking before bedtime may keep you awake longer.

3) Unhealthy diet
-Excess of
Trans fat food: fried foods, cakes, biscuits, frozen pizzas, baked goods like muffins.

Food high in cholesterol like offal, eggs, dairy products from full or reduced fat milk.
Burgers, too much red meat, whipped cream, fake spreads (buy real butter!)
Too much wine or other alcoholic drinks. [26]

-Additives and preservatives.

The main issue is their presence in almost everything you buy that is not fresh or not from a locally produced. Having a look at what is written on the back of the packet can help you understand your food better.

The most common toxins you should avoid are the following.

Aspartame or E951, is a neurotoxin and a carcinogenic sweetener present in the sugar free and diet foods. It can enhance chronic fatigue, emotional disorders such as depression, severe anxiety, and diseases like diabetes, Parkinson's, and Alzheimer's, etc.

Monosodium Glutamate or MSG / E621 kills your cells by overstimulation. Their regular consumption is related to fatigue, depression, eye issues, etc. [27]

Sodium nitrite/nitrate is another toxic preservative used to preserve packaged meat products. It enhances the red colouration and makes it look fresh to eat even if it is out of date.

Choose your local butcher as opposed to supermarkets as it can be hard to tell what you are really eating! What you put in your mouth can either benefit or be detrimental to your health. Everything is interconnected. You are what you eat! Improving your diet helps regulate your brain chemistry, improves your feeling of well-being and gives you a healthy appearance as well.

Seeking nutritionist advice and/or adopting new dietary habits is a great way to start feeling good.

B. BRAIN TRICKS TO HELP YOU CHANGE YOUR DIETARY HABITS

When you try to NOT eat something, the first thing you will do is to eat or think about 'that thing'. If you tell yourself that you don't want to smoke anymore you will keep smoking anyway unless you express an earnest desire to improve your health habits. Why does it work this way?

Geek fact: Your brain doesn't know the difference between negatives and positives. Marisa Peer, Leading Celebrity Therapist and Hypnotherapist Trainer, best-selling author, and motivational Speaker explains that it doesn't matter what you consciously wish or don't wish. Your mind takes the information and accepts it. She says, *'your mind ... does not care if what you tell it is right or wrong, good or bad, true or false, helpful or very unhelpful - it just lets it in'*. [28] 'Avoiding' something is hard because you focus on the thing you want to avoid becoming fixated with it rather than finding a solution. Suggesting something else to your brain works better.

Every time you know you 'shouldn't eat/do something', suggest to your brain a healthier alternative without using any negation in your proposition.

C. THE BRAIN'S FRIENDS AND GOOD HABITS

1) Your brain loves water, hot water

A small percentage loss of water in the brain can affect its functions. [29] Drinking hot water isn't only an old Chinese culture but it is has great benefits on your body as well. It dilates the blood vessels, which improves the absorption and hydration of the system, and helps you think faster!

✎ Accept the 10 DAY CHALLENGE: DRINK AT LEAST 1.5L PER DAY (see end of this chapter).

- Shift work,
- Reduced Daytime light exposure (people confined in offices),
- Increased Night time exposure which corresponds to screen exposure. The blue light emitted by technological devices triggers the same process as natural light. Therefore, scrolling on social media or watching a movie before bedtime delays the release of melatonin in your system.
- DST (Daylight Saving Time). It's when the government decides to add or remove an hour's sleep.
- Bad habits: irregular sleep pattern (see the sleep pattern challenge sheet), and
- Eating at irregular hours.

If you can identify with one or more of these trigger elements, find a positive possible alternative and repeat the new habits to start enjoying the results.

What happens when the clock is disturbed

The consequences depend on the person and the frequency of time shifts.

- DST can have more effects on a person who is frequently stressed and sleep deprived than someone who feels good and well-balanced.
- Jet lag isn't normally a big issue but can take longer to recover from if you are tired or sick.
- Shift work is hard on your body especially if it changes every week.
- Irregular bedtimes, irregular and unhealthy meals disturb the internal clocks of your body which unevenly releases the main hormones involved in the sleep process.

Your body needs time to adjust and if the time shifts are too numerous, your body doesn't have enough power to cope with the demand. It will result in extra fatigue. This is why adopting a healthy routine, wherever possible, is essential to being well-balanced.

Accept the 10 day sleep pattern challenge (see end of this chapter).

A study on mice shows that skipping breakfast affects the balance of their circadian rhythm, causes a loss of energy and makes them look sick. In comparison, the mice eating regularly appear perfectly healthy. [33] Grazing like a cow doesn't help either as it keeps a high level of insulin in the body (diabetic risk factor) and disrupts your normal meal pattern. Your body loses its ability to recognise when to eat.

These imbalances affect your mood and level of energy level which respond to low frequencies and vibrations influencing your thoughts, feelings and behaviour. Everything is connected: habits and gut, gut and brain, emotions, thought, actions.

The consequences of asynchrony in the circadian rhythm.

1. Delayed sleep-wake phase disorder (DSP)
This sleep disturbance is characterized by a 2 hours delay or more in comparison to others. This rhythm doesn't match with the social and working demands. These people will fall asleep due to exhaustion, struggle getting out of bed, or have difficulties dealing with the external world due to daytime sleepiness, fatigue and lack of energy.

2. Advanced Sleep-Wake Phase or 'early bird' circadian clock.
This corresponds to very early bedtimes: 6pm or 7pm.

As a result, waking in the morning is very early too (long before 6am). Sleepiness occurs in the late afternoon and when interacting with others you have difficulty remaining focused.

These people will miss hours of sleep but keep waking up early which causes chronic sleep deprivation. The other problem relies on the concern that they're not like everybody else. This feeling makes them adjust their rhythm with others instead of listening to their body. Staying awake involves using stimulating options. The consequence is a massive decrease in the quality of your sleep.

3. Irregular sleep-wake rhythm
In this case, nothing is regulated or synchronized. It is very common for people suffering from dementia or brain disorders.
The brain and body are not able to maintain a proper flow of hormones in the body. They can appear over energetic at times when they should sleep, and lethargic when they should be active. This pattern leads to exhaustion in the long run. It can appear like a nervous breakdown (depression, negative thoughts, anxiety, dizziness, insomnia, hallucinations, extreme mood swings, unexplained outbursts, panic attacks, etc.). [35]

How can you handle asynchrony of the circadian rhythm?

Firstly, identify if your situation requires medical advice and visit a doctor if needed or if in any doubt.
Secondly, look at your daily routine and review the weak points (bedtime, meals, break times, etc.).

Fill in the BASICS CHECKLIST at the end of this chapter.

Thirdly, you don't have to be like the others! A good routine is one that makes you feel good.

Consider the following advice to develop new good habits.

Taking a nap.
Opinions differ about this subject but you should simply use your common sense. If you drive or do activities that require your attention, take a nap beforehand.

Have a light dinner
Eating too much uses more energy and can lead to indigestion and bloated feeling. Choose a warm soup as opposed to a burger, some greens and fish as opposed to red meat and pasta with a mountain of cheddar on it.

Eat at regular hours. Irregular meals disturb the good balance of insulin release in your body (diabetic factor, circadian rhythm disturbed).

Late afternoon green tea or coffee are diuretic and stimulate your brain activity which you don't need when you go to bed. Choose a **hot chocolate** or **infusion** without caffeine instead.

Banish screens from your bedroom!

Accept the challenges at this end of this chapter!

THE BASICS CHECKLIST SHEET

ATMOSPHERE

1. Is there a TV in your bedroom? If yes why?

2. Where is your phone when you sleep? If it is in your bedroom, is the flight mode button on? If no why?

3. How clean and tidy is your room? 0 (a disgrace) to 10 (perfect).

4. Is the temperature in your room between 16 and 19 degrees? Adjust it to the right temperature.

5. Are there mirrors in your bedroom? Remove them.

6. Are there windows in your bedroom? Close the curtains if they are behind the bed and open the door to let some fresh air in every day if you don't have any.

7. What colours are present in your room? Add some yin chi to soothe the atmosphere if needed.

8. What is the intensity of the light in your bedroom? Adjust it if it is too strong.

9. Do you listen to your body? Go to bed when you are tired. Don't wait!

SLEEPING GEAR

11. Is your mattress too hard, just right, too soft? Change it if necessary.

12. Is your pillow too big, perfect, too low? Adjust for your neck.

SHOWER

13. Do you shower everyday? When do you shower? Practise a meditative shower everyday to relax and cleanse your body.

SPORT

14. Do you do a sport? If no, start now!

15. Do you ever rest from work and sport? If no, plan it in your routine.

HOW YOU PROTECT YOUR BRAIN

16. Do you drink enough water?

Check the smell and colour of your urine.

Malodorous and dark yellow = dehydration. Odour-free and very clear yellow = good job.

Do you drink at least 1.5L per day? If no, do the WATER CHALLENGE below.

17. Do you have a brain-friendly diet?

Do your ever eat greens, blueberries, food rich in proteins, or other healthy nutrients? If no, add them to your diet everyday.

18. How often do you eat western food?

Do you drink alcohol or caffeinated drinks and how often? Consider reducing the quantity if you 'need them' everyday or consume them in excess (more than 1 or 2 glasses of alcohol, 2 coffees a day).

19. If you **smoke**, do you smoke before bedtime? If yes, consider a healthier alternative before bedtime.

20- Do you take any **drugs**? If you are highly dependent and struggling to reduce the dose then please see a professional.

21 - If you practise a sport exposing your head to injuries, do you have regular checks? If no, just do it!

CIRCADIAN RYTHM

22- Do you go to bed at the same time everyday?

23- Do you wake up at the same time everyday?

24- Do you sleep the same amount of time everyday?
Do the sleep timing challenge below.

25- Do you have breakfasts? At regular hours? What about lunch and dinner? Write down your habits in a diary and challenge yourself with regular new habits.

26- Do you eat snacks? Have more consistent main meals if you graze too much or seek medical advice.

10 DAY WATER CHALLENGE SHEET

The aim of this challenge is to develop the habit of drinking enough water everyday and avoid dehydration.

1. Circle YES or NO everyday. If you don't manage one day, add an extra day to your challenge.

2. Write down this new challenge on your pyramid sheet if you succeed.

<u>DAY</u> 1   1.5L YES NO   Physical activity YES NO   How many litres did you drink? …. L.

<u>DAY</u> 2   1.5L YES NO   Physical activity YES NO   How many litres did you drink? …. L.

<u>DAY</u> 3   1.5L YES NO   Physical activity YES NO   How many litres did you drink? …. L.

<u>DAY</u> 4   1.5L YES NO   Physical activity YES NO   How many litres did you drink? …. L.

<u>DAY</u> 5   1.5L YES NO   Physical activity YES NO   How many litres did you drink? …. L.

<u>DAY</u> 6   1.5L YES NO   Physical activity YES NO   How many litres did you drink? …. L.

<u>DAY</u> 7   1.5L YES NO   Physical activity YES NO   How many litres did you drink? …. L.

<u>DAY</u> 8   1.5L YES NO   Physical activity YES NO   How many litres did you drink? …. L.

<u>DAY</u> 9   1.5L YES NO   Physical activity YES NO   How many litres did you drink? …. L.

<u>DAY</u> 10   1.5L YES NO   Physical activity YES NO   How many litres did you drink? …. L.

10 DAY SLEEP PATTERN CHALLENGE SHEET

If you don't sleep enough, go to bed too late or at irregular hours, this challenge is for you! This will teach you a new bed time routine. Your body likes consistency. So discipline yourself with good habits.

1. Write down your old habits, the ones you want, and what you manage to do.
If you don't manage one day add an extra day to your challenge.

2. Write down this new challenge on your pyramid sheet if you succeed.

	OLD TIME habits	NEW TIME wanted	TIME MANAGED
	MORNING EVENING	MORNING EVENING	MORNING EVENING
DAY 1	Example 7am – 1 am	6.30 am – 11 pm	Midnight – 7 am
DAY 2	Example 8am – can't tell	7am – 11 pm	7am – 11 pm
DAY 3			
DAY 4			
DAY 5			
DAY 6			
DAY 7			
DAY 8			
DAY 9			
DAY 10			
…			

IN A NUTSHELL

- Everything is interconnected; your brain, your body, and your mind.

- Unbalance in one area creates unbalance in another. Your job is to reach a good body homeostasis.

- The first steps are to reduce useless stress by creating simple new habits that can make a difference in your quality of life and sleep.

- Electronic devices are toxic elements you must keep away from your bed. They cut you off from your real environment.

- Try keeping your living space clean and tidy.

- A hot evening shower one to two hours before bedtime enhances a better sleep onset.

- A regular physical activity brings you 'feel good hormones' and keeps you fit and healthy.

- Treat yourself to a good mattress and pillow.

- Cultivate Feng Sui to attract good vibes in your home.

- Protect and feed your brain with care. It controls everything you need to live a decent life.

- The best time to go to bed is when you are tired or at regular hours.

- Your internal body clock is your circadian rhythm. It needs to be regulated with good habits and enough light to ensure a good flow of the hormones in your body.

- Melatonin is the 'Sleeping Hormone' of the body and is produced at night-time.

"I wake up every day and think,
I'm breathing! It's a good day."
EVE ENSLER

CHAPTER 6
YOUR ANCHOR FOR LIFE

Breathing is the essence of life. It is your anchor and all you have and own until you leave this world.

At birth, you cry to kick start your lungs and breathe on your own. If you don't breathe you don't get oxygen, the cells in your brain die, you cannot think, and you cannot move. Breathing is essential to living. Breathing properly and using the proper techniques are beneficial for a good night's sleep.

> *'When the breath is irregular, the mind is also unsteady,*
> *but when the breath is still, so is the mind'.*
> HATHAYOGAPRADIPIKA

I. GENERAL INFORMATION

Learning how to control your breath benefits your health.
It reinforces your diaphragm functions, teaches your lungs to absorb more oxygen, and therefore revitalizes your entire body. It improves your ability to focus and relax. It calms the mind because you learn to focus on your breath only and not on external distractions (life's hassles for example). Certain breathing techniques calm the central nervous system. As a matter of fact, a body properly oxygenated holds less tension and functions better.

Breathing exercises start the relaxation process your body needs to fall asleep. It consists of heart rate drops, decrease in body temperature, muscle relaxation, and other adjustments.
When your body slows down, it sends signals to your brain that it is time to sleep.

In this chapter, I offer some breathing exercises and personalised techniques I learnt from Reiki, Yoga, osteopathic teachings and. life experiences. You may be familiar with some of them as they mostly use the same principles. You need to practise your breathing exercises regularly (everyday preferably) to get benefits from them. I suggest you try them in the order that is written in this book to get more results if you are not used to breathing techniques. You will understand why as you go.

II. BREATHING TECHNIQUES

1. Breathing Awareness Technique

- You can do this exercise whenever you feel the need to relax.

- The purpose of this technique is to bring awareness to your breathing habits and show you how important it is. It can reveal your abilities or difficulties in holding your breath, but it is not the main purpose of the exercise. How do you breathe? Is your breathing even? Do you sometimes stop breathing? (When you carry heavy objects for example).

- This technique will calm you down as you keep repeating it.

***

1. Sit somewhere comfortable and start breathing normally through your nose.
2. After three normal breaths, take a deep breath in through the nose and hold on for as long as you can.
3. When you cannot handle it anymore (don't wait to collapse either), breathe out and go back to normal breathing.

Notice how it feels when you can finally bring some air into your lungs. It's good to breathe, isn't it? What a relief!

4. Repeat two times or three times until you start feeling some sort of pleasant emptiness or fatigue.

2. Belly Breathing Technique

- You can do this exercise whenever you feel the need to relax and feel more grounded; before bedtime for example.

- Belly breathing or diaphragmatic breathing reinforces the strength of your diaphragm, your core stability and teaches you to 'breathe with your belly'. As your diaphragm gets stronger, it does its job more efficiently and the way you breathe become more beneficial for your body.

There are different ways to do a belly breathing exercise but all consist on focusing on breathing with your belly and keeping your chest as still as possible. The following technique is part of the 'yogic breathing' practice called Pranayama. 'Prana' means – life, force, and 'ayama' means -extend. It is the formal practice of controlling the physiology of the body, i.e the breath. [1]

It may be difficult to keep your chest still as most people only breathe with their chest but with a bit of time it will become easy. Remember repetition is key to memorizing something new. If you feel good and are in a good mood, you can use the following pre-technique part to bring more serenity and power to your technique. If you feel stressed and impatient, go straight to the technique.

Let's get started!

When you empty the bottle, the liquid/breathe out leaves the bottle from the top (chest), and the liquid left at the bottom of the bottle (belly) leaves last. Logical, isn't it?

So, you should breathe the following way: **1. Your belly – 2. Your chest - and empty the air from 3. Your chest- 4. Your belly.**

Bottle breathing can be quite challenging to integrate as you have been breathing another way your entire life. Luckily, you now know the right way.

***

1. Take a seat or lie down somewhere comfortable. Straighten your back but don't force anything. You should feel calm and relaxed.
2. Place one hand on your belly at the level of your navel and the other hand on your chest, at the same level as your sternum, just under your collarbone.
Close your eyes. Start breathing normally.
3. Start noticing how you breathe. How does the air feel like through your nose? When you breathe in, notice that the air is a bit cold in your nose. When you breathe out, notice that the air feels a bit warmer this time. Then, start to notice and feel how the air gets in and out of your belly, then your lungs.
4. Let your thoughts pass by one after the other like you would contemplate waves breaking on the beach. You won't see the same waves anymore. Be aware of your thoughts without attaching any special emotion except joy and peace. You are here, breathing and it calms your mind. Smile.

~ Technique ~

Now, you are going to focus on your breath.

1. As you breathe in, notice where the air goes first. Is it in your chest or your belly? As you breathe out, notice how the air goes out first. Does it leave your belly or your chest first?

2. Take a slow and deep breath and bring the air in your belly. Make your stomach rise. Try to push away your left hand with your belly.
Keep breathing in and let the air fill your chest and push away your right hand.

3. As you breathe out, apply a gentle 'pressure' with your hand on your chest. Once the air is gone, apply a gentle pressure on your belly with your left hand to expel the air of your belly.

4. Keep breathing this way for at least 5 minutes.

5. Whenever you are ready, come back to your normal breathing, open your eyes if they were closed and be grateful for this moment.

4. 4-4-8 Breathing Technique

- You can do this exercise before going to bed or whenever you feel tense and need to calm your thoughts (overthinking, anger, stress).
- This technique helps you focus and relax. It gives you a notion of timing by bringing more regularity and rhythm to the way you breathe.

~ Technique ~

Start the same way as the previous exercise if you enjoyed it but rest your hands on your knees or on each side of your body if you are lying down. (3)

1. Start breathing in for 4 seconds, hold your breath in for 4 seconds, and slowly breathe out for 8 seconds. Take your time. There is no rush.

2. Repeat the 4-4-8 pattern or 3-3-6 if the first option is too long. Everybody works at their own pace.

3. Keep breathing this way for at least 5 minutes.

4. Whenever you are ready, come back to your normal breathing, open your eyes if they were closed and be grateful for this moment.

5. Pursed-Lip Breathing Technique

You can do this exercise whenever you feel the need to relax, to reoxygenate your body, or as part as your morning routine for example. The main purpose of this technique is to improve your lung function. This exercise brings more oxygen to your lungs and the rest of your body. Repeating this exercise everyday can have amazing results on your capacity to relax, to breathe properly, and on your ability to focus. It is an excellent exercise for everybody and especially for people suffering from shortness of breath or any other medical condition that involves breathing difficulties such asthma or bronchitis. According to Medical News Today post, this exercise might trigger tightness in your chest, shortness of breath, cough, increased mucus production, or a wheeze. The regular practice of this exercise will reduce those effects. (4-5)

How does it work?

It involves breathing a certain way which consists of changing the pace of your breath by resisting the expulsion of the air during your exhale. Your airways and chest are under 'pressure' because of the air trapped in your body. By pursing your lips and breathing out, you force out the air which is trapped through your mouth and delay its expulsion. As you breathe out slower with an element of resistance (lips pursed), it modifies the pressure in the airways and 'keeps the airways in the lungs open for longer'. . Therefore, your body has more time to absorb the oxygen.

This technique focuses on your exhale and teaches you to get rid of more stale air.

~ Technique ~

Start the same way as the previous exercise if you enjoyed it. You can put your hands on your belly and chest, let them rest on your knees, or on each side of your body if you are lying down.

1. Inhale through the nose, bring the air in your belly first, and then fill in your chest.

2. Exhale through the mouth with the lips pursed (like when you blow on your tea because it is too hot to drink) and expel the air from your chest, then your belly.

3. Inhale again through your nose and bring the air in your belly first then allow the air to get in your chest. Breathe out.

4. On the next breath, breathe in for 4 seconds and exhale with the lips pursed for 8 seconds.

You can try 3 and 6 if the rhythm suits you better. Some pursed-lips techniques suggest 2 seconds inhale but it is up to you.

2 seconds seems to be really short and can stimulates you instead of slowing you down.

5. Repeat the exercise for 5 minutes at least.

6. Whenever you are ready, come back to your normal breathing, open your eyes if they were closed, and be grateful for this moment.

6. Ujjayi Pranamaya or Victorious Breath Technique [6]

You can do this exercise before going to bed, whenever you feel tense and need to calm your thoughts, or in preparation for meditation. This is another Yogic type of breathing technique.

The specific benefits of this technique are to slow down the rhythm of your breath, to regulate it, to improve your inner strength and power, and to bring a better connection for deep meditation purposes. The technique consists of using your throat like when you fog up a window when you want to write something on it. Let's say 'Haaaa'. When you are frustrated with someone, you naturally reproduce this sound at the back of your throat. You don't exhale though the nose, but the throat, the mouth closed.

~ Technique ~

1. Sit with your back straight to stay alert and tall. Rest your hands on your knees or lap, palms down. You may close your eyes.
2. Start with a couple of deep breathes in and out.
3. As you breathe out, close your mouth and partially close your glottis to create a gentle 'Haaa' sound. It is said to sounds like 'the waves of the ocean'.
4. The second concept in the technique is to keep the same count on both breaths, the slower and longer, the better. You can start with a 4 seconds breathe in– 4 seconds breathe out and progress to a 8 seconds with more experience.
5. Practise this exercise for a least 5 minutes and come back to a few deep breaths before finishing. Be grateful for this practice. Namaste.

There are so many varieties of breathing techniques to choose from but the final outcome is always the same. A breathing technique teaches to control your breath and improves your respiratory system functions.

III. 10 DAY CHALLENGE BREATHING EXERCISE

1. On a scale of 0 (easy) to 10 (hard) rate the level of difficulty of the technique. Record it each time and notice how it changes.

2. Notice your ability to relax, to focus and how you sleep. Notice before and after the challenge if they improve.

	Technique (ex: Bottle Technique)	Length (ex: 10 min)	Before Emotions/Sensation (ex: stress, angry)	After Emotions/Sensation (ex: more relaxed, less angry)
Day 1		Min		
Day 2		Min		
Day 3		Min		
Day 4		Min		
Day 5		Min		
Day 6		Min		
Day 7		Min		
Day 8		Min		
Day 9		Min		
Day 10		Min		

3. Once you succeeded in this new challenge you can add it to your pyramid (3.Taking action and 6. Consistency Tools). It is the first part of your victory. The real success consists of keeping up with a daily practice (morning or bedtime routine).

IN A NUTSHELL

• Breathing is your anchor. It keeps you grounded and alive.

• Breathing exercises practised on a daily basis will teach you how to control your breath and will highly benefit your health.

• The Awareness Technique reminds you of the power of breathing and calms you down.

• Belly Breathing reinforces your diaphragm, teaches you how to use your belly to breathe, and keeps you grounded.

• Bottle Breathing shows you the physiological way to provide your body with the oxygen it deserves.

• 4-4-8 Breathing Technique improves your ability to focus, calms the mind, soothes and regulates the pace of your breathe.

• Pursed-lip Breathing improves your lung function, relaxes you, and helps you focus better.

• Ijjayi Pranamaya or Victorious Breath is a Yogic practice that brings you serenity, prepares for meditation, and deepens your inner strength and connection to the Universe.

• Remember that repetition is part of the key to meeting Mr Sandman. It is the strategy ingredient you must adopt to make any new learning become a habit. So practise at least one technique everyday to get results.

• Succeeding in the different challenges is a first and small step to improving the quality of your sleep. But the secret relies more in keeping up with the new habits and tips that are beneficial to you. You can report your successful challenges in your pyramid to keep them in mind.

"Laughter has no foreign accent."
PAUL LOWNEY

CHAPTER 7
THE ART OF LAUGHING

Why write about laughter? Because people underestimate its magic. Humans are so busy crying, playing victim, judging, or criticizing that it leaves less place for laughs. Although, it is an easy thing to do and it acts instantly with the only side effect of being contagious.If we could replace all the complaints with smiles, laughs, and kindness, people would be so much happier.

As you know if you have read the foreword, I was born in France. This country is not only known for its good food, red wine, art and expressive people, but also for its sense of humour and famous comedians such as Frank Dubosc, Gad Elmaleh, Coluche, Florence Foresti, and many others.

My dad used to say that laughing is the best medicine in the world. It works like magic. It has this ability to put you in a certain state of euphoria and nothing else can compete with its power. It helps you release tension trapped in your body to allow more peace. It is a perfect remedy. When you are frazzled by your routine, one of the only things capable of shifting this energy in the wink of an eye is a good burst of laughter. It is as good because of its holistic and natural way to immediately make you feel better.

'Research has shown that laughing for 2 minutes is just as healthy as a 20 minutes jog. So now I'm sitting in the park laughing at all the joggers.' [1]
UNKNOWN

I. WHY IS LAUGHING SO GOOD

According to the 'Ancient and healthy: The science of laughter' published in 2017 by Tim Newman in Medical News Today, laughter triggers the release of endorphins in the brain. [2]
Remember that endorphins are 'feel-good' hormones which naturally makes you feel happy. It increases the feeling of euphoria and is a great natural pain killer. Endorphins reduce stress and therefore promote a better sleep onset.

Laughing disconnects you from the external sources of worry or problem you may have in life. A simple giggle can shift your mood and exuberant laughter can relax your entire body because it involves the contraction of a large amount of muscles. Sometimes, you laugh so much that you forget the reason why you laughed which shows you that laughter disconnects you from a certain state of mind to enter another one closer to happiness.

Japanese researchers proved that laughing increases the release of melatonin (sleeping hormone') like the sunlight does. [3]
Laughing is contagious. The chances of communicating your state of euphoria to the person next to you are pretty high.

The article 'Laughter releases 'feel good hormones' to promote social bonding' by Honor Whiteman and published in Medical News Today in 2017, says that social laughter creates more bond with people. The more endorphins people are producing, the more laughter they can trigger within a group. Laughing with the person you live with may improve your relationship in a certain way that it promotes stronger bonds. [4]

II. SLEEP DISORDERS AND LAUGHTER THERAPY

Healthination published an article in 2011 about a study on more than 100 participants who were suffering from sleep disorders. One group enjoyed a laughter therapy and the other was a control group.

The results proved laughter had a significant positive impact on their sleep pattern and that 'casual laughter could yield[s] similar results'. [5]

In 2011, the Geriatrics published an article on an experiment about the effect of a laughter therapy on 109 people.
They targeted their quality of sleep and life, cognitive function states, and depression levels. One group followed a laughter therapy and the other was a control group. The results proved that laughing could improve their conditions after 4 weeks therapy of only one session per week. So imagine, what laughing everyday can do. [6]

I believe the ability to laugh is a habit, a sort of skill you develop and that some people develop more than others due to their environment. We actually don't laugh much at the joke itself, but at the surprise. It is the unexpected detail that triggers a reaction. Something might not be funny, but the way it sounds or looks like is peculiar and catches your attention. So you can make anybody laugh. Your reaction will depend on your habits and system of beliefs.

We all know someone who laughs easily and someone who has trouble with self-mockery or never laughs. Ask yourself with which person do you enjoy spending your time with the most? The happy one of course. So choose your surroundings well if you want to bring more sunshine into your life.
Last but not least, learn to laugh at yourself. Self-mockery reminds you that not everything is really serious.
The importance you put on things is your personal perception, not the reality everybody shares. So, laugh as much as you can without holding it in. Besides, it is an effortless workout for your abdominals.

III. WHAT ABOUT SMILING

Smile while you still have teeth!
Smiling triggers the release of 'feel-good' hormones (endorphins, dopamine, and serotonin) as well. It is communicative as you are more willing to talk to a smiling person than an angry one. It is contagious and you look more attractive when you smile (in theory). Your smile may change someone's day or life and expresses unconditional kindness which is one the most beautiful gifts life can offer. [7] Meditate on this!

Watch a comedy show before going to bed, read funny stories, spend time with happy and funny people more than with stressed and negative ones, and never forget to smile every day. Enjoy making people laugh to emphasize your positive vibes. Communicate with a smile because everything become easier to obtain and it's more beautiful this way. Anger and provocation close the door.

Try Laughing Yoga
The principle is to force yourself to laugh (in group) until the situation become so ridiculous that you start laughing about the situation.

IV. EVERYDAY CHALLENGE - LAUGH CHECKLIST

1. Write down a **list of your laughter triggers** and leave it on your bedside table. Read it when you go to bed.
2. Ask yourself everyday, **'Did I laugh today?'**
3. Think about the **last 3 times you laughed or smiled** when you go to bed and write them down in your journal. You can count and visualize the people that smiled at you everyday as well.
4. Remember your **best bursts of laughter** ever.
5. Write down this new tool on your pyramid.

IN A NUTSHELL

• Laughing is free, acts instantly, and relaxes you.

• It is natural, holistic, and powerful. It makes your body release endorphins and melatonin which are essential to regulate your sleep pattern.

• Laughter reinforces bonds between people because of its contagious ability to communicate good vibes.

• Laughter therapies have scientifically proved their positive impacts on many people suffering from sleep disorders and mental health conditions.

• Smiling is a good remedy as well. Always smile, you can breathe.

• Check the everyday challenge to bring a smile to your face and remind yourself your life isn't that bad.

"The more grateful I am, the more beauty I see."

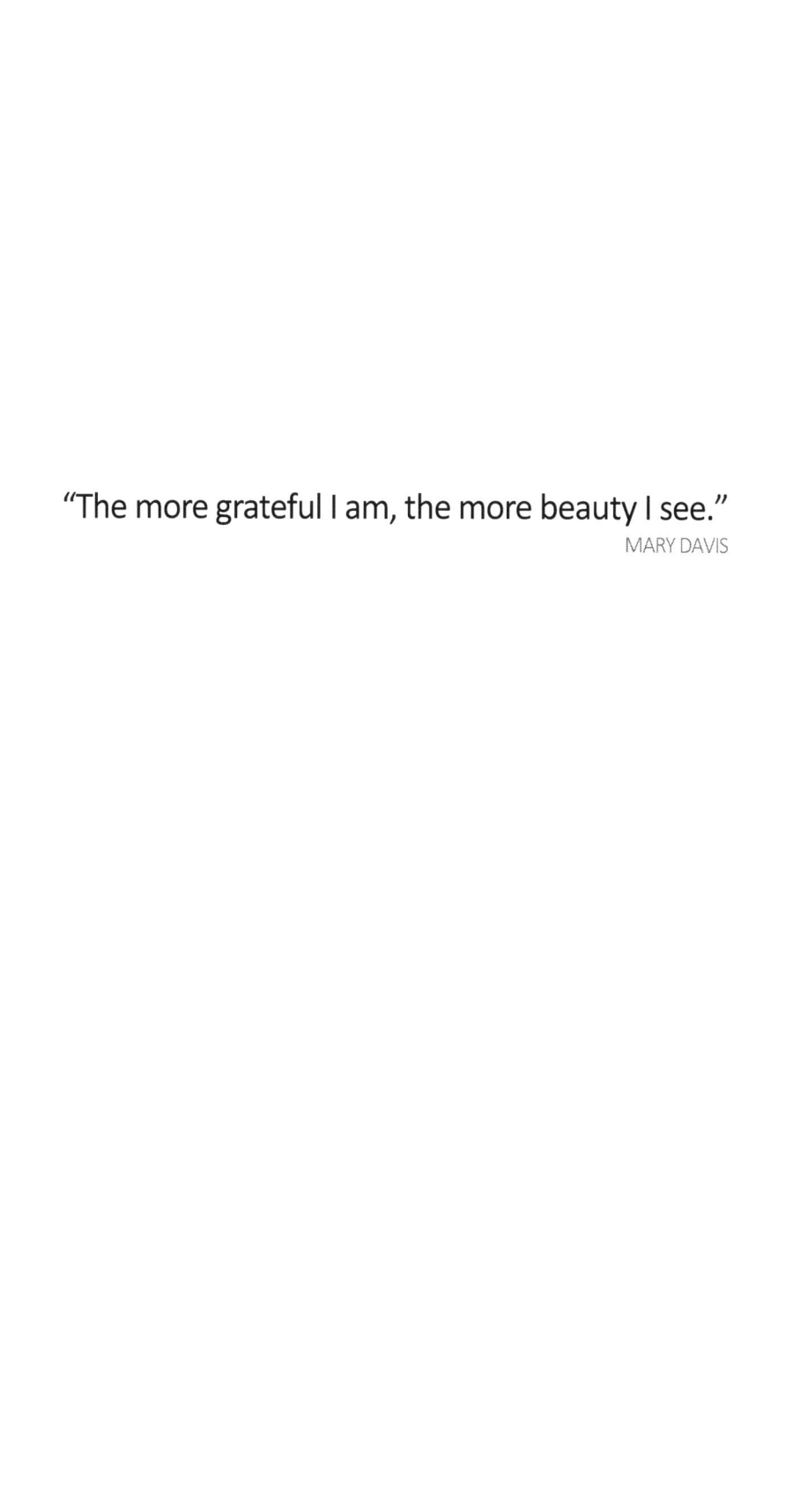

MARY DAVIS

CHAPTER 8
GRATITUDE

Do you think rich people are the happiest on the planet? Do you appreciate what you have? Do you say thank you sometimes? I am not talking about manners 'please, thank you', but about a sincere and meaningful thank you.

Being genuinely capable of gratitude is a great quality. I have been practising gratitude for about three years now and I am so happy that one of my friends and Reiki practice make me feel this way.

I. INTRODUCTION TO GRATITUDE

1. Write down these two words on a piece of paper.
Thank you.

2. Then write it down again and this time, add a very simple or obvious thing you are grateful for.
Example: Thank you that I can have a warm shower everyday.

3. Lastly, imagine how it would feel like if you didn't have that thing.
Example: What if I couldn't shower for 3 days in row?
Well, I bet you wouldn't feel confident dating after that…
The point is here to make you understand that, **you always have something to be grateful for**, as tiny as it can be and as bad as your day can be.
Don't take what you have for granted.

Maybe it wasn't there 10 years ago, and it might disappear tomorrow. It doesn't mean you have to live in fear of losing what you have or love, but appreciate what you have.

Starting to feel good, especially if you are depressed, is not going to happen in one day. Happiness is a state of mind you need to cultivate day after day until it becomes your way of life. Start saying thank you for the smallest things first because they are obvious and easy to find. It will help you focus on positive elements. Most people mainly see and think about their own problems. They talk about them more than they express their joy and gratitude for the things they have. When you are grateful for small things it emphasizes the joy you feel about all the things you already have. It helps you realize that your life is good. Saying thank you brings you more reasons to be grateful by the simple law of attraction working (chapter 3). Gratitude is the seed you need to grow to keep your positive energy at a high level, and a happy mindset which is the gateway to any achievement in life.

II. WHAT DOES A GRATITUDE JOURNAL LOOK LIKE?

Once you start writing, you may start feeling better for a few minutes or hours. It can became your daily happiness routine in a very short time. I started sleeping better very quickly after beginning my bedtime gratitude routine. Though, on certain days, I thought it wasn't enough just writing a list of thank you for this and that. You need to be grateful in a 'certain way' to get more benefit from it. The certain way I experienced was very simple but powerful.

1. After meditating, thinking and meeting people all around the world, I recalled that I had heard, 'do what you do with love and passion or don't do anything at all'. I turned it upside down and came to the conclusion that it wasn't only about love, but about emotions. When you bring an emotion to something, it all becomes more meaningful. So, I decided to **focus more on the emotions** related to the things I was grateful for and things improved.

2. Later, as I was watching *The American Dream* show by Gad Elmaleh, one word hit me, **'emphasize'**. A part of his show talks about the difficulties French people have learning English. What he noticed was that you need to emphasize. That is. 'Where to put the stress on the correct syllable. His show isn't about gratitude but he made me laugh so much that I remember this word and recalled on his 'more than happy' joke in the scene. So, I started to **emphasize** - exaggerate my gratitude emotions and it worked well too.

3. If you remember about the myelination process, the more you do something the easier it becomes to repeat it. It is the same with emotions. The more you experience a certain emotion, the easier it is to feel it again because you know how it feels.
I remember about one of those bad days when I was traveling in August 2019. I didn't feel like writing a gratitude journal at all.
I didn't even have the will to cry to release my emotions. All was blank in my mind and I hated this feeling but I wrote in my gratitude journal anyway. Nothing happened until I ran out of ink. My first thought was 'S***! I don't even have enough ink to get my sh** together!' Then, I started laughing at myself because I realized I had written ten pages. There were a lot of reasons to be grateful for.

4. I came to the conclusion that you must discipline yourself to get results especially when you 'don't feel like it' because you may surprise yourself. **Still do it anyway and something will come to the surface.** It might be an event, a smile, a hug, or just the simple realization that you are extremely lucky to have at least ten pages to write down your gratitude.
Saying thank you when you feel good brings even more power to your emotions because you already are in the positive

frequencies and all you need to do is to emphasize. But doing it when you are not in the mood enables you to shift your energy and may change your day. So say thank you no matter what.

5. Use your five senses to add details to make it more real and intense.
Example: Thank you for this warm shower. It was so good!
And I felt so great and so relaxed! I showered in a campground at 6pm, and I could hear the birds singing and the kids laughing outside. I felt cheerful. Plus, I could smell this awesome new shampoo I'd bought yesterday. It smells like coconut! I love it! Etc.
It looks cheesy but it works. Imagine yourself eating a lemon for a few seconds, and you will start salivating.

So, practise gratitude everyday no matter what, emphasize your emotions, add sensorial details, and enjoy the results.

III. POWER OF GRATITUDE ON OUR BRAIN

Studies found that people writing a gratitude journal everyday could change their state of mind.
An article published by Harvard medical school highlights the effect of a regular gratitude practice on people. This article mentions that 'Gratitude helps people feel more positive emotions, relish good experiences, improve their health, deal with adversity, and build strong relationships'. [1]

Dr Robert A. Emmons and Dr. Michael E. McCullough have led the researches about this impact gratitude has on people.
They organized the study in three groups. For weeks, the first group wrote daily complaints and unhappy aspects of their life whereas the second group wrote about happy events and thankfulness. The last group was writing about any sort of past events (positive or negative). They found out that after 10 weeks the first group who was working on gratitude had become more optimistic in their life. They felt better and didn't need to visit a doctor as much as the other groups.

Another study showed amazing results within 411 participants. They recorded high 'happiness scores' and long lasting effect of the experience on the participants. They have been asked to write weekly gratitude letters to thank someone they hadn't had the opportunity to. For the most sceptical minds those studies involved people all around the world (different background, culture, religion, health conditions). The outcome was always the same. The positive impact on the brain is undeniable.

Gratitude creates links and pathways in your brain that relate to positivity. Saying thank you everyday has an impact on your brain chemistry. [2] Emily Fletcher, founder of Ziva Meditation, published in one of her blog posts on one of the chemistry effects of gratitude on your brain. She says that 'thanks every day can increase production of serotonin and dopamine' which are brain chemicals called neurotransmitters. [3]

A neurotransmitter is a chemical in the brain responsible for neurotransmission. In other words it allows a message to pass through one cell/neuron to another. [4] Each neurotransmitter has its own function and importance on the brain and body. Some of them are regulating your sleep. Therefore, if an excess or deficiency of their level exists/persists, your sleep can be disturbed. The two neurotransmitters mentioned above are involved in the sleep regulation process.

Dopamine regulates the mood and is released when you feel pleasure and satisfaction. It helps you focus, controls the voluntary movements of the body and regulates your level of energy, mood, and libido. A deficiency leads to chronic fatigue, poor ability to focus on anything, difficulty finding any sort of pleasure, and poor libido. Patients suffering from Parkinson's disease present low levels of dopamine.

Serotonin is the happiness molecule responsible for your good mood and libido. A deficiency can result in depressive symptoms, affective disorders, negativity, low self-esteem, digestive disorders, and insomnia.

Serotonin and dopamine are not the only brain chemicals involved in your sleep pattern regulation.
ACTH (Acetylcholine) regulates certain activities in the brain associated with arousal, memory, learning, and motivation. A low level results in a lack of focus and memory (Alzheimer's patient).
GABA or gamma-amino butyric acid allows you to relax by switching off the button that activates your brain during the day. A deficiency results in a constant 'on' position that makes you feel under pressure. You can present heart palpitations, cold hands, panic attacks, anxiety, or feel overstressed/whelmed which results in finding it really hard to relax when you go to bed.

Remember this simple concept we saw in the holistic approach to the body (chapter 5). If one element is imbalanced, the adnexa will be disturbed as well, and your job is to bring more balance in your life by adopting healthy habits. You can regulate the level of your brain chemical with different methods and gratitude is one of them. It is an easy and natural way to operate. You can change your brain chemistry by changing the way you think, and therefore act. (5-6)

Practise gratitude everyday until it becomes a habit. It will create new pathways in your brain that leads to experiencing happiness more often. (7)

Another way is to have an appropriate diet. Eating what your brain needs. Protecting it to allow it to do a good job.
You already have a few notions about what your brain needs and doesn't need (chapter 5).

Dr Eric Braverman, American author, physician and medical director of PATH Medical /coordinator of clinical research for PATH Foundation NY, developed a test to discover which neurotransmitters are dominant or deficient in your brain.

The test is based on symptoms and brings subjective results only. There is currently no proven scientific test to measure the exact amount of those chemicals in the brain. [8] You will find more about it in his book *The Edge Effect*. I won't describe his research any further but it might be an incredible tool to support you. You can find it online, but I suggest you seek medical advice first, especially if you have a medical condition.

IV. 21 DAY CHALLENGE GRATITUDE JOURNAL
Exercice 1
1. Write down 5 things you are grateful for every evening before going to bed. You can divide the challenge and do it morning and evening. Set an alarm on your phone as a reminder.
2. Add it to your pyramid and keep practising until it become part of your morning or bedtime routine.

Exercice 2
1. Write down on paper what you are grateful for.
2. Ask yourself how it would be or feel if you do not have this thing or person.
3. Emphasize the emotion related to what you are grateful for.
4. Add sensorial details.

V. GRATITUDE LETTER
1. WRITE A GRATITUDE LETTER TO SOMEONE EVERY WEEK FOR THREE WEEKS.
If possible, pass this letter on. It confirms your gratitude act, the acceptance of your feelings, and gives you a sense of achievement.
If you write for someone who is not there send it the way you want to or burn it. Burning is a symbolic act that can help you let go of things more easily.

2. SAY THANK YOU TO SOMEONE WHO HURT YOU.

It will help you let go of the situation and see what you learn from this experience. Take your time to write it and remember to add details. Burn it. Take a deep breath in and out. Say thank you. You don't need this pain anymore. Let it go.

3. WRITE A GRATITUDE LIST OF THE THINGS YOU HAVE IN LIFE AND THAT YOU TAKE FOR GRANTED.

IN A NUTSHELL

- Gratitude is a powerful emotion and quality. It is a state of mind.

- You always have something to be grateful for.

- Never take anything for granted. Appreciating what you have puts you in the position to receive more of the positive seeds you grow.
It reinforces the Law of Attraction.

- Writing a daily gratitude journal makes you focus on the positives.

- Practising thankfulness is even more powerful when you emphasize your emotions, write it all down and add sensorial details.

- Studies show that practising gratitude everyday changes your mindset into a more positive one that benefits all aspects of your life.

- Daily gratitude impacts on your brain chemistry. It regulates the level of the hormones that are essential for the regulation of your sleep pattern.

- A balanced diet, and healthy habits help regulate the brain chemistry and therefore your sleep pattern and feelings.

- Say thank you everyday and happiness will follow.

"Instead of worrying about what you cannot control,
shift your energy to what you can create."

ROY T. BENNETT, THE LIGHT IN THE HEART

CHAPTER 9
POSITIVE MINDSET

"Inner happiness ... is the fuel of success".
DR JOHN HAGELIN

Many people like reading meditative or inspiring quotes about life. It gives you a few minutes of joy, hope, or consciousness. But most of the time you think, 'yes that is so true', and it might change your mood but often it is back to normal and you start acting as if you had never read this affirmation.

During my travels, I met many people who admired that I was travelling abroad on my own. I always felt honoured that I was a source of inspiration for them, but for me it was meant to be.
I was just focusing on my journey and not allowing anything to hold me back. So what is the point I want to make here? The point is that we all think a certain way and act according to our thoughts. Something is easy to do for you because you are comfortable with it. And something which isn't easy to do for you will become easy, with some practice, because you think it is possible to change the situation, and therefore you will act upon this belief and make it happen no matter what.

I. NEUROSCIENCE AND INNER STRENGTH

Marisa Peer says in her blog posts called *'make the unfamiliar familiar'* and *'Rules of the Mind',* how the brain works and its tendency to stick to easiness. Your brain likes comfort and will go back to its tendency and what it knows first anyway. (1-2) So, going away from home would be a whole new world for those people I met and an effort or a potential danger on a 'brain side point of view'. Your brain is very stubborn and always pushes you towards what you know. Marisa Peer explains that it works this way because its 'job is to keep you alive'. So, if you are used to live in a certain place and feel safe where you are, there is no reason to change it. It feels comfortable this way and your brain doesn't care if it makes you happy because you are alive and this is all that matters.

It works 'the same' for affirmations. They are positives most of the time and what it might mean to your brain 'Wow, what is it to be happy and positive? Hang on a minute... I love this concept but I don't know about this new idea.' So, as your brain doesn't know how to deal with what is different/new, it will make you keep your old and bad habits.

This **natural instinct / brain tendency** can explain why people stick to where they are and why their attempt to change their life by reading affirmations, or making resolutions for the New Year don't work.

Then, there is our 'mindset' or in other words our inner strength. It is the unlimited power we have and that can make the difference. Our mindset is the ability to believe that we can change ourselves; our behaviours, qualities, opinions, etc. We are defined by a unique life pattern made of experiences, beliefs, habits, actions, thoughts, emotions, etc.

Psychologists talk about 'fixed mindset' when someone thinks he cannot change those traits, and 'growth mindset' when he thinks it is possible to transform and develop them as much as we want. (3)

Your mindset is the element you can act on to take control over your natural tendencies, change your life pattern, and make a difference in your life. Changing your mindset requires you to be aware of your situation, to understand yourself, and to be willing enough to change your situation. Sounds familiar? Have a look back on the 6 precious stones (chapter 3) to get a better idea of the kind of mindset you stick to, or look at your pyramid.

***

As I kept travelling and discovering new cultures, new people, something came up; the most beautiful smiles on my photos were of children. Have you noticed how happy they are compared to adults? We think the way we think because we have been taught to think this way. Our mindset is the result of our education and experiences in life. We have been conditioned to think a certain way. Our behaviour and decisions are **the results of our brain tendency and mindset** which we have lived with. A fixed mindset tends to be a negative one because you don't believe it is possible to change this version of yourself .Fixed ideas close the door to opportunities that may improve your life.

Growing up with people who maintain or have a fixed mindset can affect you by manifesting your own negativity that you can become attached to.

It is a hard job to realize what kind of bubble we are living in because this is the only thing we know. If you are used to failure, sadness, loneliness, sleep disorders, being financially broke, but found a way to survive until now, then your brain thinks that 'it's okay'. So there is no reason to 'make an effort' and step into a new world to try to change the situation. And if you spend time with passive people complaining, criticising, and staying where they are, you will stick to your fixed mindset. We were born with a growth mindset and it changed with our environment. Maybe you dreamt of being a singer when you were a kid but your parents told you that it was almost impossible to succeed in this field without money, chance, and very hard work, etc. So your true desire vanished in 5 minutes just because you decided to believe someone else's opinion in a few minutes. A child is naïve and this is acceptable because he needs examples and education to grow up. Though parents and family often transfer their way of thinking on children who believe everything they hear. This can lead to young people giving up their dreams or acting out in negative ways.

Our education and experiences can lead to a fixed mindset in many fields and our job is to change our fixed mindset into a growth and positive one that allows us to achieve anything we'd like. The positive mindset is the '**you can do it**!'

II. HOW CAN YOU CHANGE YOUR MINDSET

Firstly, you must be willing to empower yourself and try different strategies to get results. If you keep doing the same thing, you will get the same results, but if you try something different you will have a different outcome. It works like mathematics. When an event reoccurs, ask yourself how you could do it differently this time (behaviour, reaction, habit).

Secondly, it is your decision to accept other people's beliefs as being yours and whether it is beneficial to you or not. Ask yourself, 'what would I do, how would I behave in this situation if I was 6 years old with my current knowledge -talent -strength?'

The answer should be, 'I would do it anyway using my adult skills/talents/strengths. The fears and judgments I hear or think about are not mine but someone else's words I heard once before. I allowed them to program my brain by accepting to let those words in. So, I don't need them anymore'.

Practise and repeat this new behaviour as much as possible until it becomes second nature and you will see results.

Some people may see positive outcomes very quickly and others may struggle a bit more. Everybody is unique and has their own background and level of motivation. Everybody has the same brain and functions. What differs is the way we use it. Your brain is a 'Matrix' you can reprogram with positive suggestion, reflection and persistence.

III. HOW TO SHIFT YOUR MINDSET TO A POSITIVE ONE?

1. DO SOME SPRING CLEANING

Clear the space from any toxic element you can identify (chapter 3). This will allow you more room to process new positive information. Remember, your brain is a computer with unlimited storage and emotions but, it can stock viruses and spams and a lot of trash. You must organize the trash stored in your system to let in some positives. You wouldn't pour red wine in a glass already full of old wine, right? If the layer of trash is thick, focus on it. One thing at time. *'Rome wasn't built in a day'.*

2. REPEAT NEW PROGRAMS (HABITS, POSITIVE SUGGESTIONS, ETC.) TO INTEGRATE THEM

- **Laugh and smile,**
- **Be grateful,**
- **Do something you love everyday,**
- **Suggest positive outcomes, repeat them by assuming they are real, and ask yourself why you succeeded,**

Asking yourself why you succeeded will force you to find the way to obtain what you want, consciously or not.

- **Surround yourself with positive people,**

It is essential you understand the impact of your environment on your behaviour. Avoid staying with negative people as much as possible. Negative people are detrimental to your health. It's like opossums in New Zealand, they look cute (if you find them cute!), but they are threat to native birds and reptiles as they compete for food sources. If you cannot avoid what is toxic for you, do something else. Stop justifying yourself! Learn to say no and don't feel guilty about it! Staying with unkind people who make you feel low or sad only cultivate negativity.

Write down a list of the people who make you feel good and explain why you like them so much.

Keep cultivating positivity everyday and spend time with people who sleep well to observe their habits. I know, you are going to say, 'yes but it's easy for them, he is rich, she is single, they don't have kids, they are not sick or they are young, etc.' but you need to be persistent and guess what, you don't know what you don't know, stop pretending you are a know-it-all about a field you suck at, and judging doesn't bring you any answers. What you call failure isn't and means you need to learn until you succeed instead.

- Cultivate kindness,
It brings peace to your mind. Criticizing people only reflects your own limitations, fears, failure and cultivates negative thoughts which you don't want when you go to bed.

> *"What isn't part of ourselves doesn't disturb us."*
> HERMANN HESS.

Find a quality you appreciate in a person that you criticize

- Learn forgiveness,
When you bear a grudge against someone, you are usually the one who suffers the most. Forgiving the others is one thing, forgiving oneself sets you free. Forgiveness shifts your mindset into a more resilient and positive way to think because you let go of emotions that disturb and don't benefit you.

- Practise visualization

It is a powerful method used to trick your brain and develop creativity, consciousness, and self-awareness. It is mostly used in meditation. It teaches you to focus the mind and disconnect from your reality. The best part of it is the possibility to imagine whatever you want to; its free style!

There is an excellent exercise that helps you rewire your brain and that many successful people practise. It consists of visualising any negative elements of your day into its opposite. Building positive memories even if they aren't real yet creates new brain pathways and connections to your system related to those positive thoughts. This process will encourage positive outcomes. As the old saying goes, 'fake it until you make it!'

Why would it work if it's not true?

You consciously know this isn't true but your subconscious doesn't know that. Your brain is made of two dimensions: your conscious and your subconscious. Your conscious is the rational part, the one that makes you think and take decisions. Your subconscious is the emotional part, the one which has no limits and keeps you alive no matter what. Your subconscious has no filter, it accepts then executes any idea your conscious mind decides to let in; good or bad, true or false. This is why feeding your brain with positive suggestions (habits, learning, affirmations, etc.) is so important to guide and inspire your creative side towards self-empowering behaviour and habits rather than the ones that close the doors to progress. [4]

In his article, 'Does your brain distinguish real from imaginary' in 2014, David R. Hamilton PhD put in evidence that no matter what you decide to let your brain think, your brain will act according to what it thinks as being there. As it doesn't know if it's real or not it will behave in order to make it happen again – 'fake again'. [5]

Many studies found that visualisation is an excellent tool to achieve ones goals. It is well-known that athletes use this technique to maintain a deep concentration and improve their performance. Dr Hamilton showed a brain scan after a 5 day study on people learning piano. One group plays, one imagines playing the same sequence, and the last one is a control group. The two first groups show the same results and the last one is blank, nothing happened. Thanks to these results and many other scientific experiments, he explains that 'what you imagine to be happening is actually happening as far as your brain is concerned'.

If you understand now that you are free to travel anywhere you want to, your brain will make it happen. Because you can imagine what you want, if you imagine yourself feeling good, smiling, laughing, and that you believe in it, your brain should release the hormones that make you feel good.

Many studies show that the brain releases chemicals during a visualization process that are the same as if the person was really acting. You probably heard of the 'love hormone' called oxytocin or molecule of attachment which is released when you express or receive love or kindness from your external world (human or pets for example). In his blog posts, Dr Hamilton reminds us about it and explains that when you visualize the same kind of act, your brain releases the same hormone as well. I haven't found the release of each hormone for all the types of visualization in the world, but if visualization works for athletes, for piano, or for love it could work for everything.

Close your eyes and visualize having a good night's sleep. Visualize that you had a great day. Visualize that you have sorted out all your hassles. Etc.

Visualization can be part of a meditation process (chapter 13), but you are not always in a mood to visualize. If your emotions interact with your desire to relax, think again and opt for other options like a running session or any other activity that calms you down.

- Practice self-love,
Learn to love yourself and accept who you are .Be grateful for the qualities you have and cultivate them. Reject any type of rejection because they are not yours. It is disguised in many forms such as bullying or any futile comment that doesn't make you feel good. If I give you a gift that you accept, it is yours, but if you refuse it is not. Just say no thank you (to yourself), I don't need it. You hear and witness but don't let it in because it is a potential poison for your mind.

- Stop watching the evening news,
This can fill your brain with negativity 95% of the time. Of course, it is good to keep yourself informed, but not about war, misery, diseases, or any sort of crises that brainwashes you with more dramas than you need before bedtime. Spend more valuable time with your relatives instead.

- You have the answer inside your head, it is cheesy but true.

IV. BAD DAY POSITIVE CHALLENGE
1. DAILY CHALLENGE SMALL HASSLES
The goal is to turn your SMALL hassles into positives.

It's a short bedtime visualisation turning your day into positives. Small hassles relate to something that disturbed your day but that you can easily handle.

For example: at work one of the customers was upset because he didn't get a discount. As you were not authorised to do it, he went mad and made you feel guilty because you know he had bought a lot of things and deserved a discount. But you are not the manager.

A positive scenario would be to ask your manager for the discount. He agrees and the customer is happy and thankful for your effort. He even compliments you on doing a good job.

As your brain doesn't know what is real or imaginary you create good memories-situations that impact positively on your brain. And when you're happy your brain releases happiness hormones which make you feel good and sleep better.

2. WEEKLY CHALLENGE BIGGER HASSLES

Same exercice as the first one but with a bigger issue.

You still work at the same place, and this time a customer has been rude to you and your manager didn't support you even though you asked for help. You feel trapped because you really need money and are too busy to find another job or too scared to apply for another job.

In this case, the situation requires more than a simple visualization; some ACTION is needed.

Firstly; y*ou can talk to your manager and explain the situation, how you feel, he will understand, apologize and make the necessary changes.*
Or you can visualize yourself, confident, preparing your resume for another position, another job with a good manager and better pay. You have the job. You are happy. You shake your new manager's hand while drinking a coffee he has just offered, and it's a sunny day.

V. DAILY POSITIVE MINDSET CHECKLIST

1. Negatives of my day into positives.
2. Any positive that happened today (from a simple smile to some great news).
3. I am grateful for (name 5 things or more).
4. I am (three compliments to yourself 3 times a day).
5. The last 3 times I laughed, smiled.
6. My affirmations about sleep:
I feel good and relaxed because ...
I had a good day because ...

I am going to have a good night because ...
I always sleep well because...
I am going to have nice and pleasant dreams because...
I will wake up tomorrow, rested and excited to start the day because...

7. The people who make me feel good are ... because ...

CHAPTER 10
PLAN TOMORROW

Obvious things such as preparing your day in advance (your lunch, getting your clothes ready), are good habits that can change the way you feel when you start the day. Being organized can be very helpful for busy people, lazy souls, night owls, or people who don't respond very well under pressure.

✎ Do you plan your days? If not, why not?
If do you, do you usually follow your plans? If not, why not?

I. 1000 REASONS TO PLAN YOUR DAY

- It reduces stress.
It doesn't take all the pressure off you may encounter but it reduces it. You are less likely to be overwhelmed by the amount of tasks you need to accomplish. If you have a hectic day approaching, you will know what to do, in which order, and things will happen more smoothly.

- It gives you some peace of mind when you wake up.
It gives you the satisfaction that you don't have to worry about the details. It is like going on a daytrip with a tour guide. I imagine that your tasks may not be comparable to enjoying a package holiday but it is the same principle.

Organisation avoids the *'OMG, I have so many things to do today, I don't even know where to start. I'd rather stay in bed.'* Sound familiar?

- It saves you energy.
You wake up with a certain amount of energy depending on how well your body was able to recover during the night. Our body works like a battery. Knowing in advance what you have to do prevents you from wasting this energy looking for what you have to do next and so on. The only thing you need to do is to read and do the task instead of hesitating or overthinking.

- It prevents you from forgetting things.

- It teaches you how to prioritize things in your life.
Organization means underlining the most important things you have to accomplish. You should try to do what is more energy-demanding first (in the morning) because this is when your stock of energy is at its peak and because it may reduce your tendency to procrastinate (famous afternoon excuses; 'I'm too tired, the shop is closed, it's not polite to call them at 6pm, etc.'). Last but not least, you won't have to experience the potential pressure you would be feeling if you weren't sorting out this tasks once and for all.

- It increases your productivity.
If you are very busy, disorganized, or procrastinate a lot, having a plan gives you more chance to accomplish your goals. Disorganized people waste time not because of the task itself but because they have to think about what they should do or not do next. Your chance to accomplish more tasks is higher because you only have to follow the schedule you wrote in advance until you get it done. It helps you discipline yourself and concentrate on your tasks.

-It brings you satisfaction
Satisfaction releases dopamine in your system which makes you feel good. Finishing what you were supposed to do usually brings this satisfaction and feeling of relief at the end of the day.

-It may give you some spare time
With a bit of practice, you will become more task-efficient, productive, relaxed, and you may be able to set some spare time aside to do more tasks or do something you like. If you think it is 'impossible' to set some free time, you may reconsider the way you use your time; for example, using lost time doing something constructive. This time can be used to read, talk to someone you love, or do anything else that makes you feel good.

II. WHAT TO DO AND WHAT TO WRITE

They are many ways to prepare a schedule but I have found this way to be helpful for the 'non-plan friendly' people (like I was). The ideas I propose in this chapter are partly inspired from the book *The End of Procrastination*, (LUDWIG, P. and SCHICKER, A.) and from my experiences, mostly. (1)

🖉 *Write down your plan on paper and place it somewhere you know you will see it (table, fridge). You can plan on your electronic device and set reminders.*

1. SET A MORNING ROUTINE

It is an essential element of your day that provides you with some extra energy and calm. It is a nourishing ritual that many successful people such as Toni Robbins, Mel Robins and Daymond John practice every day.

> *'[W]in the morning to win the day'.*
> TIM FERRISS

The purpose of a morning routine is to empower yourself with good thoughts and vibes. This good energy you get from it helps you cope better with any event that may happen in the day because you feel more at peace with your thoughts. It makes you focus on what is important. Mel Robins stresses the importance of setting priorities in the morning. One of her 'must do' tips is to not have her phone in the bedroom.

The purpose is to stop wasting your time thinking about what other people do or have, as this tends to slow you down because of your natural tendency to always compare your life to others'. Looking at what others do or have can sometimes make you feel like you're not good enough, not worthy, or unlucky.

On the contrary, cutting yourself from distractions at least in the morning (social Medias upon awakening) will help you focus on your real goals and use your energy for yourself. [2]

- YOU CAN START YOUR MORNING ROUTINE WITH A GRATITUDE LIST OR A JOURNAL.

- DO SOMETHING YOU LOVE

It is an activity that makes you grow. Would you rather wake up to take a flight to Bora Bora or go to work (even if you like your job)?

✏ What do you love? What would you love to do first when you wake up every morning?

It can be sport, music, meditation, a warm and meditative shower, writing a gratitude journal, reading, etc.

The extra plus is to go to bed knowing that tomorrow will start with something you like. You fall asleep with a smile on your face and a feeling of excitement.

'But, I don't have time to do what I love in the morning...' - Yes, you do. Wake up on time and try do what you usually do faster or wake up a few minutes earlier. All you need is 10 minutes for a start, then 20 minutes. 30 minutes to one hour for yourself would be ideal but it depends on what is possible.

Give yourself some time to reach this target and keep enjoying the process as always.

- HAVE A HEALTHY BREAKFAST
Your brain needs food to work, so treat it with care when you wake up and you will enjoy the results. For example, go for some oats, fresh fruits, Greek yogurt, chia seeds, hot tea with lemon and honey, or a good avocado on toast, etc. (chapter 5, what your brain likes).

2. WRITE DOWN WHAT YOU NEED TO DO

- **Set your priorities** instead of trying to do everything at once.
- **Start with what you really don't want to do**, so that it is done and you don't need to think about it anymore.
- **Organize some breaks** in your schedule to get some fresh air, stretch, or enjoy a smoothie instead of spending 7 hours staring at your laptop while drinking energy drinks full of sugar and additives.
- If your schedule looks good and you think nothing needs to be changed, **try something new** to fight off any potential boredom.
- **Plan less** than what you have to do to increase your chances of reaching your targets and to avoid frustration.
- If you feel creative, **customize your schedule**. It helps you enjoy the process of planning your day.
- **Don't add too many details**, it is meant to be written quickly.

III. PLAN TOMORROW CHECKLIST

1. Tell yourself, **'Tomorrow I will wake up and I will know what to do. '**

2. Prepare your lunch in advance and the clothes you will be wearing if you work.

3. Write down your morning routine if it is the first time you are doing it and add it to your pyramid. For example,

~ **Everyday, I wake up at 6am and drink a glass of water.**

~ Everyday, I write my gratitude for at least 5 things or 5 minutes.

~ Everyday, after saying thank you, I practise visualisation (what I want my day to be like, the emotions I want to experience, etc.) for 10 minutes, or go running for 20 minutes.

~ Everyday, I have a healthy breakfast (avocado on toast, fresh home-made orange juice, hot water and pressed lemon).

4. Plan the following day

- Your priorities or things you don't want to do.
- The others tasks
- Break time
- Meals
- Hobbies

Set up your work priorities if it is of any help. Smile.

IN A NUTSHELL

• Organising your day may
- Reduce stress and avoid the morning panic which can lead you to procrastinate or feel overwhelmed.
- Save your energy and guide you.
- Increase your productivity
- Make time for yourself

• Set up a morning routine to 'win the day' and try stick to it.

Your turn!

"Without Music, Life Would Be A Mistake"
FRIEDRICH NIETZSCHE

CHAPTER 11
MUSIC THE CONDUCTOR OF YOUR NIGHT

"You know what music is? God's little reminder there's something else behind us in this Universe; harmonic connection between all living beings, everywhere, even the stars."
ROBIN WILLIAMS

I. GENERAL INFORMATION

According to the National Sleep Foundation, music has many positive effects on your health. It gathers people and reinforces bonds between them. It is what makes people feel and brings consciousness to your body. You can express yourself through music and let go of your worries, anger, fears, or simply share and communicate your happiness and love to the world. Playing an instrument is even more powerful than just listening to the music because it allows you to express your emotions and heal yourself. It comes from deep within and the vibrations released by the instrument resonate within your entire body.

The article Music and Health from Harvard Men's Watch, published in 2011, explains a study led on 45 patients in intensive care and recovering from a heart attack. They found out that a 20 minutes music trial could drop heart rates. The benefits on the system remained one hour after the exposure to the music.

It helped slow down the body functions which is an essential step to ensure a good sleep onset. So, listening to some relaxing music every evening before bedtime can help you sleep better, and decrease stress and anxiety. (1)

II. WATER AND BRAINWAVE FACTS

Have you ever thought about listening to your favourite playlist or singer to relax? If not, start doing it tonight because it is the laziest and easiest way to improve your quality of sleep. Although, you may keep in mind that some music genres can relax you more than others such as jazz, classical, folk, and many blues tunes. Most of these styles of music are 'slow tunes' ('60-80 Beats per Minute - frequency)'. The frequency corresponds to the number of vibrations recorded per seconds. The fewer vibrations the lower the frequency. It is an important detail because if affects your brain and body differently.

Music impacts on our nervous system. (2)
The cells in your brain talk to each other thanks to electrical pulses. To communicate, they need chemical particles called neurotransmitters, and they need to be in tune. The cells in your brain have to be synchronised and work on a certain frequency to be able to transmit signals. Their 'synchronized electrical pulses' create the brainwaves. These brainwaves are activity related. Slow waves relate to slow frequency, moves, dreams, and fatigue, whereas the high frequency ones refer to more stimulating situations such as working or running. (3)

Different sorts of brainwaves exist. Scientists have identified the delta waves, theta waves, alpha waves, beta waves and gamma waves (chapter 2). Each of those represents a certain state of arousal and activity.

Delta and Theta are slow waves.
- **Delta** (5-3 Hz) brainwaves are 'deeply penetrating, like a drumbeat'.

They occur while we deeply meditate, during 'dreamless sleep', profound sleep, and when no contact is made with the external world. Those waves trigger the deep restorative process which is essential for the body. Delta waves are predominant in stages three and four of a sleep cycle.

- **Theta** (3-8 Hz) brainwaves are present during deep sleep and deep meditation. They are considered a 'gateway' to access hidden, lost, and unconscious information (fears, unsolved issues), but also knowledge and aptitude to learn new data.
Dr Joe Dispenza, researcher, author and international lecturer, says that your body is 'asleep, but the mind is awake'. Theta waves are predominant in stage two of a sleep cycle. [4]

- **Alpha** (8-12 Hz) and **beta** (12-38 Hz), tune higher frequencies and dominate our everyday life. They refer to our alertness and arousal state. The alpha waves correspond to the stage one of the sleep cycle. It is a light meditative state but you still stay alert. According to the blog post 'Playing Your Brain's Symphony: Staying in Tune by Dr. Joe Dispenza, it is the gate allowing you to redirect your conscious mind to your subconscious.

- **Gamma** (38-42 Hz) waves are special and pitch the highest frequencies recorder. They would 'modulate perception and consciousness.'

As you know now, everything is interconnected. So, if slow moves induce slow brainwaves, then slow waves/low frequency can induce slow moves too (fatigue, relaxation). The goal is to use music as a tool to make the cells vibrate at a certain frequency which corresponds to the 'cruising mode brainwaves'. If we use slow sound waves to push the brainwaves to tune with the same frequency we listen to, we may generate the alpha, theta, or delta brainwaves waves that correspond to certain meditation or sleeping state. In other words, emitting low frequency sound would push the brain waves to synchronize near the same frequency. Therefore it would encourage the body to rest and catch some Zs.

As many other studies show, an article from NCBI called 'The impact of music on the bioelectrical oscillations of the brain' published in 2018, proved sound waves could impact on brainwaves pattern. (5)

Michael J. Breus, PhD, DABSM published on The Sleep Doctor™ an article in 2018 about 'Binaural beats: an old sound for better sleep?' (6) The articles highlight the effects of sound waves on brainwaves. He mentions that 'at certain frequencies' brainwaves manage to 'align with those frequencies'. Which means that listening to a certain frequency could induce the same frequency of vibration in the cells of the body.

More experiments have been done and more studies need to be led in this field as well, but this is one of the examples that scientifically explain the benefits of music on our health.

***

I believe that everybody has his own experience and perception of life and that music impacts differently on each brain.

The situation is more complex than a simple question of tuning same frequencies together which slow down the system.

Our emotions and living atmosphere matter and hold specific vibrations as well.

Dr Masaru Emoto, Japanese scientist and famous water researcher, explains the effect of the environment on the structure of water. Why talking about water? Because this is the main element of our body. (7)

His results explains that the shape of the crystal water is different according to the music genre it has been exposed to. Classical music generates harmonious and beautiful photographs whereas heavy metal tunes change the structure of the crystal into a chaotic and unhealthy appearance. The results are similar when the water is exposed to a loving, kind, or grateful atmosphere compared to hatred or evil feelings. In other words, listening to aggressive sounds (black metal for example) and lyrics praising negative thoughts or emotions such as hate, sadness, or anger can disturb the harmony of the structure of the water into your body. Our thoughts, our emotions, the words we use hold a vibration that water can resonate with, and by extension, that our body can sense.

III. WHEN TO LISTEN

As mentioned in the chapter gratitude and positivity, the more positives you bring into your life, the better your body responds. Music has therapeutic effects on your psyche because it can trigger emotions you may need to release.

There are two reasons why you should choose your playlist smartly. Firstly, it's always better to fall asleep with a smile on your face than with puffy eyes. Secondly, you cannot consciously control where the external information (music vibrations) go when you sleep.

Our brain is bombarded with a million bits of information everyday but we are aware of only a few of them. Our subconscious plays the role of a powerful filter by allowing it to let only the important data go through. This helps your brain focus on the important things and prevents it from wasting too much energy trying to process a massive amount of useless data. Eventually, your subconscious let your conscious mind deal with less data (prioritizing, making decision, etc.). [8] The fact is, your conscious mind isn't operating when you sleep which doesn't allow you to know or control what is happening to you. You are at the mercy of your subconscious mood. As you fall asleep you enter alpha, then theta waves (stages 1 and 2) which are the gateway to your subconscious and the good timing to process new information for better results. Your brain becomes an open door to positive and negative suggestions you cannot control to let in or not consciously. Your subconscious will respond to these suggestions (music vibrations, lyrics, affirmations, movies) according to your beliefs, to your brain natural tendencies, and it may not be what you would consciously agree to let in. This is why it is essential you pick up good tune frequencies and positive suggestions before bedtime. Therefore, you should listen to the music that resonates within you and makes you drowsy, euphoric, and peaceful. No matter what relationship you have with music, always keep in mind the magic it triggers in you.

Create your playlist of slow and cheerful tunes and enjoy it when it's bedtime.

IN A NUTSHELL

• Music reinforces social bonds, brings about body awareness, and helps   release negative emotions.

• Some music genres benefit you more than others because they affect your body differently.

• Music impacts on our nervous system. The cells in our brain communicate thanks to chemical particles which need to be in tune to transmit information. Their synchronisation create brainwaves.

• These brainwaves are related to our state of activity and arousal. Beta waves are present when being alert, delta and theta while we sleep, and alpha is when we feel drowsy (morning, bedtime).

• We can use music to synchronize the frequency of our brainwaves with the tunes we listen to.

• Dr. Emoto Masaru demonstrated the effect of the environment on the structure of crystals water. Listening to harmonious music and loving thoughts can create healthy crystal waters unlike heavy metal or negative suggestions.

• The music genre and words you listen to hold certain vibrations that induce healthy crystal patterns or not.

• Our body is mostly made of water which is vital to help you understand that listening to gentle and cheerful music cultivates and keeps your body healthy.

• When we fall asleep, we enter alpha, then theta waves. Those waves open the door to our subconscious mind which behaves according to our beliefs and natural brain tendency. It is essential to suggest positive words and harmonious tunes as you fall asleep.

"Until one has loved an animal,
A part of one's soul remains unawaken."
ANATOLE FRANCE

CHAPTER 12
THE POWER OF NATURE

Mother Nature is the purest source of energy you can find. If you don't live in the middle of a forest you can always walk in a park, buy yourself a small fountain, a bonsai tree or any other plant you fancy. Trees transform the CO_2 around you into the oxygen you need to breathe. This is a little reminder that you can always find a way to enjoy the simple treasures our planet has to offer and that can help you feel better.

I. NATURAL REMEDIES VS TRADITIONAL MEDICINE

Sleeping tabs may help you but in the short term only. Relying on a chemical component to sleep creates bad habits and a certain difficulty weaning yourself off it. The repetitive use of medication can deteriorate the function of an organ in your body.

If your diet consists mainly of processed food, sugar, additives energy drinks and you take medication, two things can happen. Firstly, you will keep overloading your body with toxins. Secondly, you will increase the amount of work your body need to provide to cope with the demand. For instance, your liver and your kidneys are vital filters for the body. They control what can go into your blood and what needs to be eliminated. The more toxins you ingest, the more these organs have to work to purify your system.

This takes up a lot of energy and eventually generates fatigue and complications. This is why it is essential to use as many natural methodologies as possible. If you think you found a natural alternative to help you sleep or feel better, talk to your doctor to find out what can be done to stop taking medication.

Always seek medical advice first before reducing your dosage or stopping any medical treatment.

II. NATURAL TIPS THAT ENHANCE A BETTER SLEEP

AFTERNOON AND EVENING TEA – INFUSION

The most common natural drink tea contain herbs that enhance relaxation and calm the nerves.

- Chamomile has sedative properties.
- Valerian calms the nerves and anxiety.
- Lime flower 'is said to lower blood pressure'. [1] Therefore, it helps the body relax.
- Vervain (contains verbenalin) soothes the nerves and helps stimulate the secretion of dopamine and serotonin.

If you remember, these are the neurotransmitters that make you feel good and this is exactly what we want. [2]

- Tincture of Lavender (or Palsy Drops). Everybody know this nice smell of lavender but you can actually consume it as an infusion. [3] (Get the edible version, of course!).

You should drink your last tea or infusion about 2 hours before bedtime as it needs to be absorbed if you don't want to wake up in the middle of the night. Certain drinks have some detoxifying or diuretic properties (green tea for example).

This book doesn't provide any medical advice. Please always ensure you do not have any possible allergy to those components. If any doubt remains, seek medical advice.

SLEEPING SCENTS OR AROMATHERAPY

Some scents have relaxing properties. You should use natural methods to diffuse the scents (avoid spray which are not eco-friendly). You can use a diffuser with natural essential oils, a few drops in hot water, or dropping lavender essential oil on your pillow for example.
One the most famous scents is lavender.

- **Lavender** helps you relax and sleep by reducing the blood pressure. [4]
- **Ylang Ylang** has good results against hypertension and depression and improves sleep quality as well.
- **Vanilla** reminds us of islands and holidays but relaxes you and enhances good mood as well.
- **Sandalwood** is very special as it 'increases theta brain' waves. If you remember, theta waves are the slow brainwaves enhancing deep meditation and sleep.
- **Jasmine** used as an infusion or as a scent calms anxiety and heart rate, promoting sleep onset.

III. CRYSTALS

Gems and crystals have become famous for their healing properties. They have been used all around the world and for many centuries B.C. Cassandra Eason explains in her book *Crystals for Love and Relationship* that 'They are useful in every aspect of daily life'. They help on a spiritual, psychological and physical aspect. As everything is connected, acting on one aspect can influence the two others. They are used for many purposes that help achieve a state of well-being. You can use crystals as jewels, elixirs or as decorations in your home or workplace.

Many studies have proved that crystals could have a measurable impact on our bodies. *Crystals are used to provide complementary support but don't replace any medication.* It is about energy, as always. Energy is vibration.

Everything that moves vibrates, and therefore creates energy. As we move, we create energy to move (ATP mitochondria). Atoms, molecules and ions constitute solids and liquids. They hold energy and are capable of motion between each other. This allows liquid to get its texture. Solids are much more compressed but get enough space for tiny movements 'which can cause vibration' - energy. In other words, a crystal can vibrate. [5]

If a crystal can vibrate, it can vibrate with our own energy as well. More studies need to be done to clarify the impact of all the crystal on the body. Though, we already know this: quartz is used for radios and computers, but it also regulates clocks and watches. They 'maintain a precise frequency standard, which helps regulate the movement of a watch or clock, thus making the timepieces very accurate'. [6]

Each crystal vibrates at a certain frequency and has specific properties. The following promote relaxation and serenity.

Amethyst and its purple soothing colours helps let go of things that don't serve you well anymore. Saying good bye frees the mind from stalling energies. The amethyst stone connects you to the divine, to your spirituality, and harmonizes your nervous system and brain. [7]

Pink or Rose quartz is called the "stone of love". It is used to help calm and clear negative emotions related to heart matters. It rebalances love-related emotions, and enhances forgiveness. Forgiveness chases away anger. Pink Quartz is a very gentle and soothing crystal you can use to bring some unconditional love in your life.

Moonstone is excellent to rebalance feminine energies and mood switches (periods, menstruation). It rebalances the crazy hormones in your body and saves your energy because overreacting or being emotionally unbalanced can be exhausting. It brings more peace of mind, although I wouldn't use it during the night as it is a powerful stone.

Celestite or 'Blue Heaven Stone' is a powerful but gentle crystal to use. It is perfect for your bedroom to enjoy its calming effects

It helps improve your lung and breathing functions. You can use it for meditation. It brings you mental clarity, serenity and enhances your spiritual and psychic side. It is a guardian angel stone. [8]

HOW TO USE THE CRYSTALS

The crystal chooses you. When you see it, hold it in your hand, and you don't want to let it go, it means that it resonates with and for you. Crystals are designed for one function at a time. As they hold a specific energy, you shouldn't use your amethyst for calming insomnias and use the same stone three days later for other purposes (example: to quit your job and start a new life). The thoughts and vibrations are different.

You need to take care of your crystals and clean them.
The main way is to wash them with spring water. Salt water may deteriorate the quality of certain stones and interfere with their properties. If you enjoy the principle of healing yourself thanks to stones, I advise you buy a book that explains what is good for each type of stone you decide to use.

Some stones like malachite absorb a lot of negative energies and it is very important to clean them every time you use them. Every few days should do the job for the other stones, but it always depends on how heavy the emotions you release are. You will feel it is time to clean them when you have no more results.

Devi Brown, author of the book *Crystal Bliss,* uses singing bowls. It is another very efficient way to clean the crystals. He mentions the use of 'Tibetan metal bowls with wooden mallets or quartz singing bowls with suede-wrapped mallets'. The vibrations emitted by the sound of the bowls get rid of unwanted energies that doesn't serve the crystal and you.

Another good way is to burn some sage (you can buy a bunch of sage). Place the crystals on top of the sage for a few seconds (not more than 3 seconds) while you place your intentions to cleanse the negative energies and ask for 'a reset' of your stone.

Do not sleep with the stones you used during the day as the energies absorbed may come back to you and don't use your night stones during daytime either for the same reasons. Most of crystals can be used together, but some of them hold special vibrations which shouldn't be mixed with others (obsidian for example).

You need to **activate your crystal** by setting your intentions and expectations from it. Be clear minded about it. (7)

For those who practice meditation, you can meditate on it and activate it this way with the crystal in your hands. For those who practise Reiki, you can send some Reiki to your crystal. It empowers the stone even more and you can cleanse it the same way. At last, for those who are unfamiliar with meditation or Reiki, just take the crystal in your hands, and close your eyes. Ask your crystal what you want it to do to support you.
Say thank you and start enjoying its benefits.

You need to re**charge** them with energy to keep them active.
Your crystal is an element that comes from a natural source: Earth. So, recharge it with a natural element. Remember to reboot your crystals regularly, especially if you use them a lot.
The best way to recharge your stone is to place it in direct sunlight for at least four or five hours or leave it outside exposed to the full moon.

Crystals are your possession and resonate with your body only and not with someone else's body. Don't let someone else touch your stone because it might interfere with the vibrations your crystal holds for you. If it happens, clean and recharge it. You may reprogram it if the person who touches it doesn't inspire much kindness. Even your best friend can transfer unconscious negative energies to your stone.

When a **stone breaks** or gets lost, it means that it has done its job and that you should stop using it. Don't try to find it by all means. Move on with another stone, and if something happens to the same crystal, it means your body may not vibrate with it anymore. Get another kind of stone that refers to other emotional needs if you enjoy the benefits of crystals or find another way to sleep better if you still have trouble sleeping.

How to dispose of it
Bury it to give it back to its original source.

IV. THE POWER OF ANIMALS

Dogs, cats, parrots and other animals, are amazing little creatures. What is fascinating about them is their innate ability to give you unconditional love. They are loyal and always happy to see you (a cat doesn't always show you its affection though).
In the United States, about 68% of the population owns a pet..[9]

Studies show that pets owner suffer less from anxiety, stress and heart diseases than non-pet owner people. For example, children raised on farms who spend their time surrounded by animals and therefore present a stronger immune system and fewer allergies than children not exposed to animals.
Animals have this power to calm you down because they behave like emotional sponges. They are empaths and have this sixth sense that allows them to feel emotions with more intensity than you do. Their presence makes you feel better and more peaceful.

More great things about pets
- They don't judge you. You don't have to argue or feel the need to justify yourself because they accept and love you anyway.
- They make you laugh which releases endorphins in your system that make you feel good.
- They keep you warm inside and outside.

- As you get attached to them, you release a love hormone called oxytocin which is another happiness molecule trigger. (10)
- If it's a dog, it makes you exercise and is a good motivation for you to stay fit and healthy.
- If it's a cat, you will probably run after it and not with it and it might control your emotions a bit too much, but its purring sound and silky hair are so irresistible that they always win the battle.

This purring sound has healing properties. (11-12)
It corresponds to a certain frequency between 25 and 100 Hertz. According to some research, this range of vibrations benefits the body in many ways.
- It would help broken bones heal. (25-50 Hertz).
- The cat purr is known to lower the level of stress hormones which prevents you from sleeping.
- It lowers the blood pressure (and therefore the risk of heart attacks) which is one of the important steps that allows to relax before bedtime.

A cat is the perfect teacher to observe if you want to learn how to breathe peacefully. It is a 'chill machine' and teaches you by mimetism how to stay calm.

Your pet costs you less than years of treatment with a psychologist. I think there are enough reasons to be pet friendly. Spend time observing it, cherish the moments with it with exaggeration, don't take it for granted, and never underestimate their 'magic'!

IN A NUTSHELL

• Medicines fill your system with toxins.

• A repetitive ingestion of sleeping tablets and other drugs combined with an unhealthy diet drains too much energy from your system and may create complications in the long term.

• Chamomile, valerian, lime flower, vervain, or tincture of lavender have healing properties that encourage relaxation and can help you sleep better.

• Jasmine, lavender, Ylang ylang, and sandalwood scents have relaxing effects on your system.

• Crystals give you complementary support to make you feel better.

• Crystals vibrate at a certain frequency that resonate with your body. They hold specific healing properties.

• You can put an amethyst under your pillow, place a celestite, a pink quartz, or a moonstone in your bedroom to sooth the atmosphere and help you sleep better.

• Each crystal is unique, personal, and requires care.

• Pets love you unconditionally, calm you down and reinforce your immune system.

• They are cheaper and may be more efficient than years of therapy with a psychologist.

• The cat purr has fascinating properties.

• Get yourself a new best friend to stay fit and-or healthy.

"When you realize there is nothing lacking, the whole world belongs to you".
LAO TZU

CHAPTER 13
MEDITATION

I. GENERAL INFORMATION

Everybody has heard about meditation or has tried it at least once in a lifetime. The number of people in the world enjoying this practice never stops increasing [1] (200 to 500 million people and probably more than that).

The idea that a lot of people have about meditation isn't always accurate. We usually think about monks in a temple meditating and chanting mantras all day. The truth is, you don't have to wear a special outfit, stay in a monastery, or sing 'A-U-M' all day long to do it. Meditation is an excellent tool for self-empowerment. It can be a simple way to relax or a real life purpose for those who want to become meditators. I believe it is a real journey that leads you to understand who you are and beyond. It is a skill you develop with practice. The definition and importance you put on the word 'meditation' changes as you evolve in your practice. Meditation and religions are two different things. You don't need to believe in any higher power to meditate, as much as you can be a believer and meditate, or use meditation within your religious practice. Meditation is accessible to anyone who wants to achieve perfection, gain wisdom, or is convinced the world has endless treasures to offer. How you meditate is related to who you are and to what you want. Grand Master Akshar, Himalayan Yogi, says that meditation is for people who believe in life and love and that it 'will decide your destination'.

Meditation can change who you are, therefore, the choices you make. It is a way to reach perfection and everybody who is willing enough has access to it at their own level of experience. (2)
The main reason why people meditate is to escape from their reality. They seek calmness and peace of mind to reduce stress and anxiety in their life.

II. MEDITATION AND' MEDITATION'

Meditation is called meditation for a reason. Laughing isn't playing drums, it is laughing, Singing isn't having a hiccup, it is singing. Meditation isn't playing tennis, it is meditation.
David B. Dillard-Wright and Ravinder Jerath write in the *Everything guide to meditation for healthy living* book that meditation is 'the stilling of all your conscious faculties in order to be present in the moment'. (3) You really meditate when you still the mind and disconnect from everything around you including your thoughts. It is the art of finding a still point in your mind that allows you to connect to higher frequencies. During meditation you should not sleep or lose control of your body. You should feel amazed because everything is amplified in its better version (4). It is like observing the delicate perfection of the Sakura which blossoms every spring in Japan. It shows its perfect pink colours and unconditional love vibrations to its surroundings.

Everybody has a certain vision and experience of life and this is why there are so many ways to meditate or should I say, to reach a 'state of meditation'. Not thinking about anything requires some practice. You may feel discouraged from trying to experience this stillness in your mind if you don't feel it immediately. If you are not familiar with it or impatient, exercising with different 'forms of meditation' will be easier and more 'seducing'. We talk about 'different forms of meditation' but remember that the real moment is when you reach stillness in your mind and think about nothing.

The different 'forms of meditation'

- Hobbies: practising a sport you enjoy help focus the mind on the exercise and game. Playing a musical instrument, reading, or go fishing are all forms of meditation that develop your concentration and calms your mind.

- Visualization Meditation creates a virtual atmosphere that makes you feel good and keeps you away from your negative routine. It can calm your nerves, give you time to restore your energy and develop your creative skills.

- Mindfulness Meditation develops self-awareness. It teaches how to enjoy the present moment without distraction. [5] Mindfulness helps increase the connectivity between 'the everything' and the nature of life. It is about observing ourselves and our surroundings to clear our minds. Observation without judgement develops understanding and acceptance of the different situations we experience in life and helps one think more objectively. A 'still unstill' mind has this ability to observe the permanent motion of the universe.

- Mantra or chanting meditation consists of repeating sounds and sequences of words to achieve calm and balance. Chant aims 'to purify your body and mind'. The sound used 'breaks up energetic blockages' because it vibrates with your body and tunes it to the frequency you emit while singing. It is a type of meditation considered as sacred in many religions and a mystical science for Yoga practice. [6]

In meditative toning, the sounds are used to make your body vibrate at the same frequency than the sound itself which refers to a certain state of awareness.

A (aah) refers to a Relaxation state,
E (aay) with acceptance,
I (eeh) with stimulation,
O (ooh) with focus,
And U (uuh) with empathy and harmony.

Mindworks describes more forms of meditation in their blog post 'What are the Different Types of Meditation?' [7]

- Focused meditation is the ability to focus the mind on one thing at a time (e.g. a cup of coffee on a table). If you lose attention, accept it and start over.

- Spiritual meditation can be practised different ways. The religious way empowers the connection between the believer and the Divine. The non-religious way develops awareness and actualization (the commitment to reach our best in everything). They develop kindness and connection.

Where can you practise?

Anywhere is possible but your aptitude to focus your mind on 'nothing' depends on your experience. For a start, you want to find a quiet and comfortable place. Practise where you can escape your everyday life – for a few minutes at least. You can meditate in a group or try guided meditations which are very popular and can help people not used to meditating to strengthen their focus.

III. MEDITATION AND HEALTH

Meditation has amazing effects on health. Some studies show that people suffering from insomnia and who started practising meditation could improve their quality of sleep by 75%, and about 60% for patients suffering from PMS (premenstrual symptoms) or anxiety. [1] You don't have to meditate three hours every day to enjoy the benefits. A ten minute routine can power boost your day and ease your nights. A daily practice can make a meaningful difference to your life.

Meditation rebalances your mind, your body and your spirit. Keeping those three elements in harmony is essential to ensure your well-being and keep your nervous system balanced.

MEDITATION

According to Dr Joe Dispenza, 'just taking daily small moments for meditation to reach this present state of mind and body, allows your nervous system to recalibrate back into harmony and balance.' (8) You can find peace of mind and relaxation, as it optimizes your ability to fall asleep easily. It teaches you to focus the mind on one thing at a time which makes you forget about your life hassles.

Meditation is a good tool to use during your introspection work and self-assessment (chapter 3 and 4) because it develops your aptitude to observe things without attaching emotions to them. So, you make better decisions and with practice, stop wasting time with situations that don't help you. It makes you anticipate and therefore readjust to your own reactions.

Once you understand the concept that nothing stays still, you know it is possible to shift your energy to a growth mindset and make better decisions. You can handle your emotions better, set your priorities and start acting consciously to save yourself time and energy. It gives you the opportunity to look at yourself differently. You are flesh and bones but also an endless source of energy because of your connection to the Universe. Life is a constant stream of interferences: fear, panic, doubt, stress guilt. They can distract you and this is why you must learn to control them. This is where meditation can perform miracles if you start practising regularly. It can ease anxiety, depression, stress, poor sleep quality or any other health issues. (6)

Using time to meditate makes you save time. And time is too precious to be wasted, so use it well (chapter 3-fuel towards action- will, priority, time, action).

Last but not least, meditating keeps you grounded and reconnects you to yourself as you concentrate on the present moment from which we are easily disconnected. Developing this ability to enjoy the 'now' helps you appreciate the joys of your life with more intensity which is a key to happiness (chapter 9).

Add Meditation to your Daily Positive Mindset Checklist.

Meditation will help you magnify everything you have and enjoy more of it (strategy-keep enjoying the process-precious stone-chapter 3).

IV. NEUROSCIENCE AND MEDITATION

Studies show that meditation boosts the flow of more than 7 of the main body chemicals; amongst them are GABA, DHEA, Growth Hormone, Melatonin, Serotonin, and Endorphins. [9]

As already mentioned, serotonin is one of the happy molecules of your body. Endorphins are the feel-good chemicals you release when you practise a physical activity, laugh or meditate, and melatonin is the sleeping hormone. [10] Researches founded 'that meditation models the brain into a natural 'deep sleepy machine'. It improves the quality of the deep REM stage, the general sleep quality, raises the level of melatonin in the blood, and enhances quicker recoveries when ill. Meditation can push the brain to enter delta, theta, and dream frequency brainwaves. Some studies show brain scans of meditating monks. They reveal their aptitude entering gamma brainwaves and reach an extreme focus state (also, they practise a lot).

The images show that mediation increases the loss of awareness with the environment (disconnection from interferences).

This state has some similarities with magic mushrooms acting on the brain. [11] If you remember, the brainwaves frequency are activity-related and correspond to specific degrees of awareness. As meditation enhances the ability to reach this state of deep meditation and relaxation, it can encourage creativity, ability to learn faster and better, and your motivation in general, which means that it can reduce your tendency to procrastinate.

Fact: Children experience more theta waves than adult and this is one of the reasons why they are great at learning anything new in a shorter time than us (example: languages). [12]

Mediation benefits to delta brainwaves which corresponds to a very deep meditation state, recovering process and link to the unconscious part of the mind. But not only. It enables you to shift brainwaves from one to another.

Dr Joe Dispenza explains that theta brainwaves are the gateway to reprogram your brain. We can say that when we start falling asleep or upon awakening, our brain is more likely to open to new information that could replace any pattern we want to get rid of in our life.

✎ Add a meditation practice to your morning routine or start practising it at least once a week for a start, and write it down on your pyramid.

V. HOW TO MEDITATE

Master Sri Akarshana explains a few important basics on meditation. He reminds us that 'Everything holds energy', so get your own yoga mat to practise. (4) Meditate only when you are at peace. You cannot do it when you are stressed because your mind is too preoccupied thinking about something. (13) You may choose some breathing exercises (belly breathing), a physical activity, or shout as loud as you can as you hide in your car (sounds funny but it really helps), if you want to calm down. There is an endless list of ways to meditate but knowing a few of them only will be enough for a start. Pick any style of meditation that makes you happy and enjoy this time which is yours.

VI. MEDITATION PRACTICES

Now that you have read the chapter 6, you should be an expert in the art of breathing...
Sit somewhere comfortable with your back straight. It is okay to feel some tension but you must be free of pain. Put your hands in a praying position your thumbs level with your heart.
This hand position called 'Anjali Mudra' is a way to honour yourself, your teacher or the universe, and focus the mind on your practice.
- As you take a deep breathe in, move your hands towards the ceiling and look at them. Breathe out and spread your arms out on each side of your body towards your feet.

- Breathe in and do the opposite move towards the ceiling, then breathe out and bring back your hands to the praying position. Repeat the move three times.
- Close your eyes. It reduces external distractions and shifts your brain into alpha frequency.

1. Simple breathing practise
- Put your hands into the Anjali position or let them rest on your knees. Palms up you are receiving energy from the universe or facing down protects your energy from outside. Choose the position that you are comfortable with.
- Then focus on your breath only. Fill your belly with air first, then your chest, then empty your chest and your belly. The goal is to focus on your breathing and to think about nothing, not even the fact that you are breathing. Regular practice will make it easier to realise. If you start thinking; it's okay, just keep practising and stay there as long as you want to.
- Take a deep breath in and out. Slowly start moving your body. Whenever you are ready open your eyes.
- Thank yourself and the universe for this practice.

2. Mindfulness meditation. Develops awareness to your body and focus on your senses.
- Start meditating the same way; sit with your back straight and your hands resting on your knees.
- Take a deep breath in and out and close your eyes.
- Bring awareness to your body. You are here. Now. Feel the presence of your head, your cheeks, your nose, your eyes, your hair, ears, and so on for the rest of your body.
- Feel your chest, your stomach and your ribs expanding when you breathe in. and your abdominals contracting when you breathe out. Scan your body from top to bottom
- Feel your sitting bones on the surface you are sitting on. They connect you to the Earth and make you feel grounded.
- Now that you have experienced the sense of touch, keep going with what you can hear, smell, taste, and see in your mind.

- Once you have concentrated on all your senses, you reach a state of relaxation and intense well-being.
- . Stay there as long as you want to.
If you start thinking, it's okay, just keep practising and breathing until you reach this still point in your mind again.
- Take a deep breath in and out. Slowly bring back your body into motion. Whenever you are ready, open your eyes.
- Thank yourself and the universe for this practice.

3. Mindfulness meditation. Focus on your body and your thoughts.

Let your thoughts come to your head. Once the story starts, let it happen for a short time, then detach yourself from it by observing it. Your job is to observe your thoughts.

For example: You start thinking about the bills you need to pay (think: **'it's okay'**), you see the numbers on the papers (**'it's okay'**), now you start experiencing some frustration (**'stop'** there and don't get into the story anymore because it is an emotion you need to step away from). Your job is now to observe. Tell yourself, '**I observe** that... - I need to pay some bills, **I observe** ...- the amount, **I observe** ... - it doesn't make me feel good. **It's okay'**. Then let another story start. If the same story happens, keep telling yourself what you observe. The word 'observe' helps you detach from your feelings because you put yourself in
the position of a story teller or a witness (and not a victim). Observing a situation or a feeling instead of experiencing it will bring more clarity of mind and help you make better decisions.

I learnt this kind of meditation from a very kind monk I met in Thailand. His teachings helped me balance my emotions many times and I hope it will help you the same way.

4. The hourglass meditation using visualization

- Start the meditation the same way as before, sitting with your back straight and your hands on your knees.
- Take a deep breath in and out and close your eyes.

- Now imagine that your body is an hourglass. The sand it holds represents all the tension you feel in your body and mind. The top of the hourglass is your head and the bottom is your feet. As the sand starts falling down so does your tension.
- Take a deep breath in and out. Feel the texture of the sand touching the inside of your face and skull. It is nice and gentle on your skin. The sand is slowly falling down, touching on its way your forehead, eyes, nose, and mouth. Every time you breathe out the sand reaches another part of your body and the previous part it just left is now free and light.
- Now it is going down on your neck, your shoulders, your chest and upper back, lower back and belly.

The top of your body feels so light you could almost fly like a balloon when it's released in the air. But you are present and you feel this grounding energy on your lower body.
- The sand leaves your pelvis, your thighs, and your legs are now free of tension.
- The sand now touches and leaves your ankles and tickles your feet. You are sitting on the top of a sand dune. Feel the sand leaving the rest of your body as you meet the ground, the Earth. You feel warm, calm, safe, light but grounded.
- You shouldn't be thinking about anything now because you are here in this very moment. If you start thinking, it's okay, just keep practising and breathing until you reach your still point again. Stay there as long as you want to.
- Take a deep breath in and out. Slowly bring back your body in to motion. Whenever you are ready, open your eyes.
- Thank yourself and the universe for this practice.

🖋 *You can practise before bedtime to relax. It takes the time you want to dedicate to it, but remember it is time for yourself.*

🖋 *You may record your voice or the voice of a happy person to use these exercises as a guided meditation.*

Happy meditation!

IN A NUTSHELL

- Meditation is an excellent tool for self-empowerment.

- The definition and importance you put on the word meditation change as you get more experience.

- Meditation brings self-awareness and self-consciousness. It changes your perception of life into a growth mindset and makes you more responsible for your life.

- It focuses the mind on the present moment and brings clarity of thoughts.

- You really meditate when you stop thinking and manage to disconnect. Meditation is: a state of stillness in your mind that allows you to enjoy the present moment.

- Meditation is a key to happiness. It relaxes you, recalibrates harmony and balance in your system, and keeps you grounded.

- Meditation and its 'forms' regulates the flow of important chemicals to your brain which are essential to sleep and feel good.

- It conditions the brain into a natural 'deep sleepy machine'.

- It pushes the brain enter delta and gamma brainwaves. So, it enables you to shift brainwaves from one to another and gives access to reprogram your brain, to dream, and recover faster.

So go get a yoga mat and start today!

"To dream is to allow our subconscious thoughts exceed our limitations"
A-LO

CHAPTER 14
DREAMS

You spend one twelfth (about 7 years) of your life time dreaming. Oneirology is a very complex and fascinating science. The greatest philosophers such as Sigmond Freud, Carl Jung, Aristotle and Saint Thomas Aquinas dedicated years of study in this field. It keeps triggering a high interest in scientists and psychologists. They try to understand the mechanisms of our dreams in the name of science, their love for discoveries, but most importantly for medical purposes.

I. THE SCIENCE OF DREAMS

When do we dream?

As you know now, our sleep cycle is made up of an average of 4 to 5 brainwaves cycles: the non REM sleep (stages 1 to 4), and the REM sleep (stage 5). The REM brainwaves are close to the waves we present when being awake. We dream in the REM stage. The body is 'paralyzed' but the brain is 'awake'. It is 'easy' to wake up a person during this paradoxal sleep and if you wake up at this stage you will likely report a dream. Then, a new cycle begins with stage one (non REM sleep). The sleep is light as well but as a new cycle of brainwaves started you probably lost and forgot your dream even if you wake up at this stage. [1]

Why do we forget or remember our dreams?

Everybody has dreams but we usually don't remember them.

We dream in non-REM sleep. Our brain works just enough to gently consolidate some information in our memory, but it isn't very active and doesn't process much emotion or sensation.

The chances of remembering our dreams at this stage are pretty thin. Then, the REM sleep occurs. The length of this stage increases as we go further in the night (5 to 40 minutes) and thus allows more time and chances to create longer stories. Besides, our brain starts being more active which allows sensations and emotions to be processed. The long-term memory involves our attention, emotions, sensations, working memory (up to 10 minutes), and a hippocampal processing step for consolidation (up to 2 years). [2] Therefore, when emotions and sensations are involved in dreams, it is easier to remember. This gives more chances to recall a dream if we wake up during the REM sleep.

Many studies have proved that sleeping is essential to the memorization process. So, why don't we 'memorize' our dreams?

The article 'The brain may actively forget during dream sleep' published by NHI reveals some studies led on mice running a battery of memory tests during REM sleep. [3] A team of Japanese and American researchers found out that a group of neurons (MCH neurons) normally known for stimulating our appetite, would also control our tendency to forget or memorize new learnings during the REM sleep. Dr Kilduff explains that their activation during the REM sleep would 'help the brain actively forget new unimportant information' by preventing the consolidation process in the hippocampus. Francis Crick, co-discoverer of the DNA double helix suggests that REM sleep (mostly) would be a good opportunity for the brain to sort and store the data.

The paradoxal sleep stage would be a filter that prevents our brain from being overloaded with useless information. So, remembering our dreams would depend on which part of the cycle we wake up, on the presence and intensity of the sensations or emotions processed, on the activation of the MCH neurons, on our state of mind, health conditions, and level of stress. Note that more studies need to be led to fully identify what controls our aptitude to remember our dreams.

What dreams represent for us

Most dictionaries agree to define dreams as a succession of stories or images occurring in our mind as we sleep. It is more complex than this simple definition of course. Even if this concept is not shared by all the researchers and philosophers, most of them state that dreams would be the expression of hidden secrets or unhealed emotions. They can also bring a solution, or even a warning about something that has passed or about to happen. Indeed, our conscious mind (decision maker) may not be willing to accept, or confess to some information because of our social boundaries and judgements, or because of our tendency to procrastinate. The problem with rejecting your responsibilities is that you hold onto blocked and toxic energies in your life. This creates too much tension in the long term and forces your brain to find solutions elsewhere. Hence, dreams seem to be a way of releasing overwhelming information. Your dreams will keep manifesting as long as you don't change your behaviour and sort out the problems. Dreams are messengers and act like a safety valve for the body.

Our frontal lobe analyses what goes through our mind and is turned off when we sleep. So we accept all sorts of stories our conscious self would probably not allow to show in normal circumstances (awake). We are not aware of who and where we are anymore. Everything is possible. We experience them with more or less intensity depending on their meaning. Dreams are classified and named differently depending on researchers but the main terms remain the same.

We talk about common dreams, lucid dreams, premonitory dreams, dreams of past lives, and post-trauma dreams. For instance, **lucid dreams** are very interesting. They occur during REM sleep and mostly between 5 and 8 am in the morning. They happen because our frontal lobe is 'abnormally' turned 'on'. This allows you to experience the dream in a normal state of mind where you can be the author which controls and changes the scenario. It is similar to intense daydreaming. (4) According to some people, lucid dreams would allow you to change the' future 'to our advantage, see ahead, or control what is going to happen. They encourage 'latent clairvoyance' and 'genuine insight.'

Why working on your dreams would help you feel and sleep better?

Firstly, nobody is going to save you and as discussed in the chapter 3, you are responsible for what happens to you. Being a victim is not an option but understanding (chapter 3, precious stone) will give you many tools to suggest positive options to improve your overall well-being.

Carl Jung and Sigmond Freud believed and tried to prove that dreams are a gateway to our subconscious. They developed the terms manifest content (story) and latent content (meaning behind the dream). According to their research dreams are here to express ourselves and reveal scenarios or symbols of any secret or deep desire. Such a process would be a natural therapy to release conscious and unconscious trouble we hold. (5)

Craig Hamilton-Parker explains in his book *The Hidden Meaning of Dreams,* that dreams enable the mind to regain harmony by evacuating information that could overwhelm us. Dreams can create disturbing and unpleasant contrasts with your reality that you cannot afford to ignore. Therefore it pushes to act. We know that releasing emotions and repetitive patterns can make you feel better. So working on your dreams will empower you.

Last but not least, dreams unleash your creative side. As your frontal lobe isn't operating, nothing (environment) not even you, will control and stop your imagination. Creation encourages neurogenesis which keeps your brain young and strong. By doing so, it facilitates the consolidation of new information.

What disturbs our dreams

- **A demanding job** which requires your permanent attention may keep your brain on alert mode all the time. This overwork supresses your ability to relax and let your subconscious express itself, therefore your capacity to dream until you get the opportunity to relax. [6]
- We think of a good **bottle of red wine** as a good idea to feel drowsy and catch some Zs. Unfortunately this can lead to the abuse of alcohol. According to the article *'How Alcohol Affects the Quality—And Quantity—Of Sleep'* published by the National sleep foundation, alcohol would change our sleep cycles regulation. It increases the presence of delta waves (non REM sleep). If the stages 1 to 4 increase in lengths, the REM sleep (stage 5) is reduced or disappears. As we mostly dream in stage 5, our dreams could be 'blocked'. Besides, as this stage is one of the most restorative sleep, its blockage can lead to sleep deprivation. [7] So, thinking that alcohol on a daily basis, can help is a big mistake as it disturbs the sleep pattern.
- According to the *'Drug and Dreams'* [8] article published in the Indian Journal of Clinical Practice in 2013, **prescriptions drugs** can disturb the regulation of our sleep cycles because of their aptitude in changing the brain chemistry (influence on the neurotransmitters). It has different sorts of consequences on our dreams. Some patients would have more nightmares, some would dream more, and others would dream less. For example, the drugs which stimulate our central nervous system (amphetamines, caffeine) would increase the quantity of dreams but not always their quality. The research led by Dr. Sarita Goyal, Jyoti Kaushal, MC Gupta, and Savita Verma, mention that 'amphetamines are associated with vivid and unpleasant dreams

whereas caffeine has been used to induce lucid dreaming, because it makes one sleep lighter.' Though sleeping lighter means that you can be awoken more easily. So coffee isn't a solution either. The most obvious conclusion is that any unnatural way to fall asleep won't really help you and things will get worse in the long run.

II. WHAT CAN WE DO ABOUT OUR DREAMS

Craig Hamilton – Parker researches mention the beliefs Yogi have about dreams; any sort of dream scenario can be modified as long as you want it to be. As we discussed (chapter 3), it is easier to act on something you understand. So analysing your dreams will enable you to act on them. You need a plan. This is the one I use and I must say it works fairly well. I hope it will help you.

FIRST STEP
Work on what can disturb your dreams (alcohol, drugs, stressing job).

SECOND STEP
Accept your dream. Don't ignore it if it feels shameful or hurtful. Doing so expresses only your fear to deal with the subject.
You need to have a growth mindset about your dreams. They are here for a reason and can serve you well. Be grateful that you are having dreams.

THIRD STEP
Understand your dream. You can either write it down in a dream journal or talk to a friend or a professional. Don't be afraid of all the details you remember because they may bring the solution to your problem.

How to understand or assess a dream

Your dreams reveal what you cannot consciously express because of your principles, beliefs, education, environment, etc. Understanding your dreams means you need to identify any detail that could lead to possible reflection work. In her book *Healing the nightmare freeing the soul,* Margaret M. Bowater talks about different types of nightmares. [9]

- She refers to life **issue nightmares**. They often are a reflection of certain events in our real life, or an accurate 'portrayal' of emotional experience. You can identify if a part of your dream refers to a 'déjà vu' situation. It can be an image showing you what you do wrong.

- Another type of dream she refers to is the **'shadow self-nightmares** '. They outline your behaviour, a trait of your personality you consciously deny.

- **Post trauma nightmares** are based on real drama. The trauma is sometimes so intense that it is too hard to handle on your own. Holding enormous emotions is dangerous. Therefore, your brain needs to find a way to release the pain for your own safety. And this is through repetitive nightmares.

Fact: Some researchers have developed the 'survivor guilt' concept. They reveal the influence that society can have on survivors. Once again it is a question of beliefs and the tendency of our society to put everything and everybody into categories (e.g. after your studies, everyone should work, get married, have children, and buy a house). In the **'survivor guilt concept'** situation, the environment of the victims usually brings more attention and kindness to the 'biggest victims' category. Although all the survivors experienced the same events, the 'luckiest' category was left behind. This triggers the feeling that their pain wasn't that important compared to others. Therefore they wouldn't have the right to feel traumatised. [10] They would then experience the event over and over again through nightmares to punish themselves for being alive because they think they don't deserve to express their pain or ask for help. This situation can last until someone listens to them and acknowledges their trauma.

This could allow the release of their terrible emotions eventually.

Many scenarios and types of dreams are possible but understanding their meaning is essential to heal. The recovery is better when the dreamer tries to understand and do something about their situation. The passive dreamer rarely heals.

ANALYSE YOUR DREAMS TO UNDERSTAND THEM

1. Write down your dreams on paper and add as many details as possible.
2. What you were thinking about last night before you fell asleep.
3. When did this dream start for the first time? Is it a recurrent dream? Write down the frequency.
4. Can you identify a relationship with your reality? If no, are you sure? Are the facts/emotions present in the dream exaggerated?
5. What sensation or emotion do you experience in your dream and when you wake up?
6. How do you behave in your dream? Are you active or passive? Are you fixing problems or creating some? Are you a victim, a trouble maker, or are you responsible?
7. Do you behave the same way in your dream and in your life?

Understanding your dreams can bring you answers about certain aspects of your life and push you to act differently. A dream can be a simple guide, or a way to release something you just managed to deal with. It can be the simple release of the last piece of the puzzle. If this disturbing dream comes back, it means you have to work on it.

FOURTH STEP
Find ways to get rid of your demons.

1. Refer to the spring cleaning and switch button questions (chapter 3).

2. Rewrite happy endings to your dream to offer an alternative option to solve the problem and read it a few times when its bed time. Example: *if you are attacked in the street, visualize you are fighting and winning (option 2).*
3. Exercise with the Daily Positive Mindset Checklist (chapter 9) and the following statement 'I always have nice dreams and I remember them because...'
4. Take more action (Chapter 3: Fuel towards action; Will, Priority, Time, Action). For example, if you are attacked in the street (in your dream), you can learn to defend yourself by starting some martial art classes for example (in the real world). You will feel active and your brain will use those new information and learning of self-defence to your advantage if you dream again about being chased or attacked. But this time, you will know how to defend yourself, you won't feel unsafe or scared anymore, and your bad dream will likely stop.

Many therapists can support you in your attempts to reduce nightmares such as sophrologists, EFT practitioners, hypnotherapists, etc. I urge you to try any natural therapy that may help you and contribute to minimize medication or drugs. But and as always, refer to a doctor if your health conditions requires special attention.

Using dreams to your advantage

- Some studies suggest that **increasing the length of your night** would naturally give more REM sleep and therefore more chances to dream. (11)
- As you have more chance to remember a dream if you **wake up during a REM sleep**, you can set up an alarm 20 to 30 minutes earlier than usual. It may interrupt your REM stage and give you a chance to remember it.
- You can **train having lucid dreams** by try solving certain situations in your life. Craig Hamilton-Parker suggests asking yourself during the day 'Is this a dream?' in order to question your subconscious about reality.

With repetition (a few weeks), your subconscious will keep asking the same question during the night. Then you can amplify the process with bedtime affirmations, 'Tonight I will have a lucid dream'. By doing so, you are anticipating the creation of a dream by telling your subconscious that you will have a dream anyway. You could condition the brain by asking how your subconscious has succeeded. Questioning your subconscious would force it finding the solution to your problem.

🖉 *Start a dream journal and ask yourself the good questions.*
🖉 *Add your dream journal to your pyramid.*

> Be the master of your dreams, not the victim.

IN A NUTSHELL

- You spend about 7 years of your life dreaming.

- We mostly have dreams during REM sleep and have more chances of remembering them if we wake up during this stage.

- The long term memory process demands our attention, sensations, emotions, working memory, and a consolidation step.

- MCH neurons in our brain would regulate the memorization process of the new learnings during REM sleep by preventing the consolidation step of the long term memory process. They would prevent our brain from being overloaded with unnecessary data.

- During our sleep, the frontal lobe is turned off. This allows our subconscious to express itself without external interferences.

- Dreams are succession of an expression of hidden secrets and unhealed emotions. They act like a safety valve for the body.

- Dreams are a gateway to our subconscious. They 'call attention to things in need of healing.

- Our sleep patterns are influenced by drugs, medicines, alcohol, and our life style. They disturb the brain chemistry and therefore our dreams.

- Handling your dreams requires a plan of action. Acceptance. Gratitude. Understanding. Cleansing and action.

- You can get rid of your demons.

Sweet dreams!

"All you need, You already Have."
SOMEONE

CHAPTER 15
THE BEAUTY OF REIKI

I. GENERAL INFORMATION

Reiki is a natural energetic healing medicine which comes from Japan and was discovered by Dr. Mikao Usui in the early 90s. It means 'rei' - spiritual, divine and 'ki' - energy, breath, or force. Today, it refers to the term 'spiritual' or 'universal energy'. I like to think about Reiki as the unconditional love we receive from the universe. [1] Reiki is accessible to anyone. The only requirement is an open-mind and the desire and acceptance to feel better. For the people who are more familiar with self-development, Reiki can go beyond your expectations and change many aspects of life. Because it 'heals at physical, emotional, and spiritual levels', it is a holistic practice and a state of mind. It refers to 5 principles therapists adopt in their everyday life and practice: For today only, let go of anger (be at peace), let go of worry (have faith), be grateful, be kind and be honest. [2]

II. HOW DOES IT WORK?

Reiki circulates through the practitioner to help rebalance the energy of the patient's body. It is an intuitive self- healing process triggered by the presence of a Reiki vector (therapist) who transfers the energy received from the external sources(human, animal, plants, crystal, events, nature, etc.) to the patient.

The practitioner plays the role of a vector. He doesn't create the energy or heal the patient directly. But through practices of mantras, symbols and meditations, he masters how to channel the energy coming from the universe to give it to the patient. The energy received pushes the body to self-healing/regulation and helps regain harmony and balance.

As the energy goes through and into the 'healer's body', it gives Reiki to the practitioner first, then goes to the patient. It can be very powerful. When you give Reiki to someone, you receive it at the same time. In other words, a Reiki practitioner heals himself while treating others.

The body decides what to do with this energy at this certain time and places it where it belongs. It only accepts what it can handle and what it needs at the time. The therapist usually recommends waiting two to three weeks between two treatments if it has been a 'heavy session' but there is no real rule. It will depend on how you deal with the situation. A daily 15 minute practice can be very beneficial as well.

For instance, if you want to receive some Reiki because you suffer from headaches, it may not stop them at first. Though, the Reiki will focus on a more important element that your body needs to deal with at this very moment of your life. This important element can be an emotion to release or the simple need to get an energy boost that helps you recover after a busy week. If you need to release an intense emotion you may need some time to adjust to the 'new you' before a possible second treatment.

III. BENEFITS OF REIKI

Reiki can have miraculous effects on your well-being.
Firstly, it is a pure and good energy that cannot harm you.
- It is well known for its relaxing and anti-stress results. Many patients fall asleep during the session because of its soporific effects.

- It can help reduce the physical tensions you suffer from (example: muscles) and improve the quality of your sleep.
- It brings you calm and serenity with regular sessions.
- It is a kick-start to push the body to rearranging itself. When your hormonal system is imbalanced, your body may struggle to find compensation. Reiki can regulate your mood and appetite (it stopped my cravings in less than a month).

You don't have to practise Reiki, but trying it often leads to adopting it. At first, Reiki training (level 1) requires 21 days of self-treatment. It works as a body and mind cleanser For example, I lost my appetite for 3 weeks, released all sorts of emotions, and slept a lot. It didn't release certain of the fears I had but it changed my perception of life in the long term. The benefits I experienced were immediate. Reiki can make you 'feel high' or euphoric. As a matter of fact, when you feel better, you go to bed in a good mood and you sleep better. Always keep in mind that it might not make you smile every time. As you release negative energies you have to let them go. You have to accept feeling them in order to let them go. You may cry, feel anxious, feel sleepy or lost for days, etc. Let it go, say thank you and move on.

IV. MORE THAN A SPIRITUAL PRACTICE

Have you ever felt tired or relaxed after visiting your physiotherapist, chiropractor or osteopath? You often sleep well for one or two nights following the treatment. Reiki produces the same effect because it moves and shifts the energies in your body. The motion of these blocked energies requires your body to adjust to the new information it has received. Integrating new data into your system can be energy sapping. Because your body has worked a certain way for a certain time, it needs a few hours, days, and even weeks to accept this new organization pattern.

Example: A somatic dysfunction (costo-vertebral joint) prevents your ribs from moving freely. This dysfunction triggers a painful breath in. If you persist with this osteopathic dysfunction your body will reorganize itself to 'hide' the pain. This adjustment may require you to use some muscles more than others which can lead to tension.

If you are not familiar with listening to your body, I want you to try this simple test; contract your biceps for 15 seconds or more, and as hard as you can.
The tension you feel while contracting your biceps is a tiny example of what your body can endure. Your body can hide and handle more fatigue than you can imagine. When your therapist releases this costo-vertebral dysfunction and helps your muscles relax, two things happen. It sets your pain free, and it lets go of all the tension you have been accumulating. As your body needs energy to readjust you will feel tired after a treatment. Reiki can trigger the same kind of reaction on the body. The release of an emotion sets free all the tension you hold and that is related to it.

Results show

The article 'Reiki Really Works: A Ground breaking Scientific Study published' by Green Lotus in 2011 explains the results of their experiment on stressed-out rats made in 2008-9. After receiving Reiki, the records showed significant improvement in their level of well-being, depression and anxiety. [3]
The medical field increasingly uses Reiki 'healers' in oncology services. The efficiency of the discipline never stops surprising doctors. For example, Dr Mehmet Oz, a cardiovascular surgeon, is famous for working with Reiki practitioners during 'open-hearted surgeries and heart transplant operations'.

An article called 'The Science Behind Reiki' by Bernadette Doran, BS, RMT was published in the Summer 2009 issue of The Reiki Times (magazine of the IARP). [4]

She explains the science behind Reiki. Krinsley D. Bengsten experimented on mice with cancer. He treated them for an hour every day for thirty days. Those without treatment died, those energy-treated lived. Their cancer went into remittance. Half of them were reinjected with the same cancer cells but the mice 'didn't take' the cancer because they had developed an immunisation against it. Others studies presented the same amazing results with about 80% of survival.

Studies have proved that the measurable electric and magnetic fields were presenting the same frequency as the one needed to 'stimulat[e] tissue repair'. It is close to the earth's magnetic field. Rollin McCraty, research director at the Institute of HeartMath, outlines that 'Compassion and loving intention amplify the magnetic field.' This explains why Reiki is sometimes called unconditional love.

Nota Bene: It is very important to have a 'good feeling' about your Reiki practitioner. There are different lineages of Reiki, different teachings and some practitioners may not be 'good' for you. Go with your gut, talk to your practitioner first, or ask someone you trust to get some recommendations.

Enjoy Reiki!

IN A NUTSHELL

• Reiki is a natural healing and holistic medicine discovered by Dr Mikao Usui in Japan in the early 90s.

• It is the universal energy accessible to everyone willing to heal.

• Reiki flows according to 5 principles which are: Let go of anger, let go of worry, be grateful, be kind and work honestly.

• The therapist is a vector who channels the energy from the universe and give it to the patient.

• The energy received encourages self-regulation and harmony research of the body. Reiki effects may be emotional, physical, and spiritual.

• Your body only takes what it needs at this specific moment of your life.

• The benefits of Reiki are numerous but the main purpose is to restore a good balance by releasing negative energies with positive frequencies.

• Electric and magnetic fields hold the same frequency which stimulate tissue repair and are influenced by our emotions. It is close to the earth magnetic field.

• Like for any other therapist, choose your Reiki healer well.
You should see them or hear their voice beforehand.

• Reiki brings you peace and a good night sleep.

> "To find health should be the object of the physician. Anyone can find disease".
>
> A.T. STILL.

CHAPTER 16
OSTEOPATHY

"An osteopath is only a human engineer, who should understand all the laws governing his engine and thereby master disease".
A. T. STILL

I. OSTEOPATHY FOR DUMMIES

Andrew Taylor Still discovered osteopathy in the last 1800s and the word 'osteopathy' was created on the 22nd of June 1874. Andrew T.S was an American surgeon, doctor, and pastor. [1-2] Osteopathy is defined as a holistic alternative medicine which uses manual techniques to help the body restore its homeostasis.

'The Unity Function [3]
The Human body does not function in separate units but only as harmonious whole.'

In order to treat the patient, the osteopath will consider the body as a whole. For example, he might release a joint in the ankle, then your knee, to unlock your hip, etc. Osteopathy is a science that studies, finds and treats the unbalanced systems of the body. It is the 'rule of the mind, matter and motion'. A.T. Still.

In other words, the osteopath considers all the areas of the body to treat and help the patient rebalance himself.

What does an osteopath treat?

The therapist can treat neck, back, shoulder, knee pains and many other joint pains. He can treat migraines, digestive problems, sleep disorders, chronic fatigue, and other ailments as long as the patient doesn't require specific medical attention beforehand. For example, if you have the flu, appendicitis, or a severe disease such as cancer, your osteopath should send you to your general practitioner or the hospital depending on the situation. Osteopathy is supposed to be a preventive medicine, but people tend to forget that prevention should be considered before the healing process. In other words, patients usually refer to an osteopath when the pain appears or gets worse.

Concept and goals of osteopathy

The concept in osteopathy is to find a coherent explanation that leads to understanding the present reason for consultation. What does the patient suffer from? Why? Which elements, 'osteopathic dysfunctions', or events are responsible for the current situation?

The goals are to help the patient feel better, to identify the cause(s) of the effect(s), and to treat it (them) in order to suppress the effects. Andrew Taylor Still explained that the body is a unit (a whole), the structure governs the function (cause and effect), and the job of the therapist is to 'find the lesion, treat it and leave it alone'. [4] The therapist uses his knowledge of anatomy, physiology and the biomechanics of the body to establish a protocol of treatment. Then, the treatment shows the way to the body and allows the possibility of reorganizing itself without blockages.

II. THE BENEFITS OF OSTEOPATHY

On a psychological aspect

An osteopath is merely considered a 'psychologist of the body'. Some emotions can be released by the simple touch or treatment of a certain part of the body. This is because the body memorizes emotions. We talk about somato-emotional reactions. [5]

We know now that emotions, words, or music hold a certain frequency of vibration (crystal water) which is energy.
A treatment can help you release emotions that have been trapped in your body (blocked energy). The motion of the structure will shift this old energy into a new one that sets the area free of negative emotions and trigger a somato-emotional response (emotion release related to the area treated). The second psychological impact is explained by the effect of the treatment on the body. Provided the results are good and if the patient feels better physically, his mental state will naturally improve as well.

On the physical side

The osteopath uses manual techniques to rebalance the areas of the body where 'osteopathic dysfunctions' exist. Releasing the tension trapped in a part of the body can - Improve the function of the structure which is affected and vice versa,
- Can increase its mobility and reduce the pain related to it,
- As a result, can improve your quality of sleep, [6]
- Can decrease chronic fatigue,
- Can increase the flexibility of the body (everything is readjusted),
- An osteopathic treatment requires the body to readjust to its new 'configuration'. This process may be energy demanding and cause some fatigue. This is why we often feel tired after manual therapeutic treatment.

III. HOW OSTEOPATHY HELPS YOU SLEEP

The innervation and circulation to an organ makes it work. If you don't bring blood to your heart, it will stop beating, and if you cut the nerves that stimulates the functions of a certain muscle, it won't contract anymore.

The osteopath can help the brain change the signal that disturbs the sleep by acting on releasing the tension that create the pain and by using techniques that regulate the central Nervous System. Pain can be the reason why you cannot fall asleep, or why you don't sleep very well. Pain is the direct or indirect consequence of a structure in the body which is not balanced anymore. When it is intense, the pain can control your brain and command it to concentrate on it instead of focusing on what makes you sleep.

- The osteopath can help the body restore the mobility of the area that triggers this tension and pain. As a reminder, the nervous system is composed of the central and peripheral system. The central system is the brain and spinal cord and the peripheral system is represented by the somatic and autonomic system. The somatic takes care of the information coming from and going to your muscles, skin, joints, etc. The autonomic system regulates the parasympathetic and sympathetic systems through the brain and spinal cord via sensory information (pain, for example). Those two systems control the stimulation or inhibition of the function of the body (the parasympathetic slows down the organs to allow digestion, rest, etc. and the sympathetic is the accelerator of the body which keeps you alert and active.). The spine is anatomically connected to the central nervous system. An osteopathic lesion can disturb the nervous system to the point of causing sleeping disorders. An osteopathic lesion on the skull, spine or sacrum influences the function of the parasympathetic and sympathetic system.

- The osteopath can help regulate the couple parasympathetic sympathetic by rebalancing the central axis; occiput (back of the skull) - spine - sacrum of your body. So, releasing the pain promotes a better quality of sleep and rebalancing the system helps regulate the nervous system responsible for the stimulation- inhibition actions regulating your sleep.

IV. WHAT HAPPENS DURING A TREATMENT

An osteopath asks questions about your pain, your medical history, your life and its main events. The answers you provide highlights the elements necessary to lead to a diagnosis.
Example: Car crash, office work on a laptop every day, noisy children, city life can trigger migraines.

These questions help the therapist assess if he can treat you or if you need to be redirected to another health professional.
Example: If he suspects you have a medical condition, he will advise you to visit your doctor for tests (X-rays, MRI, blood check, etc.).

An osteopath is not an obstetrician. Observing your skin, your profile type and your body is part of the examination. He gets information from his observation that helps find a treatment or redirects you to another professional depending on your needs. The therapist may ask you to move in certain positions, breathe deeply, cough, move your eyes, or contract some muscles to allow certain techniques to be performed.An osteopathic treatment requires a good knowledge of the body, practice turned into a skill, and an Indiana Jones mindset (finding the treasure - the cause).

V. YOUR RESPONSIBILITY

Most people expect miracles from a treatment. In order to feel better, it is essential to work as a team with your practitioner. The truth is that a therapist has the information you may need to feel better but if you don't listen, act, and follow his advice, you won't feel better.

Remember that it is always up to you and that blaming someone else for not taking your responsibilities won't help you. So, help yourself with a good attitude.

IN A NUTSHELL

- Osteopathy is a holistic alternative medicine which uses manual techniques to help the body restore its homeostasis.

- In order to treat the patient, the osteopath considers the body as a whole.

- An osteopath can treat a wide range of ailments as long as the patient doesn't require any special medical attention beforehand.

- The concept in osteopathy is to find a coherent explanation that leads to understanding the present reasons for consultation and establish a protocol of treatment.

- The goals are to help the patient feel better, identify the cause and treat it, and let the body heal itself.

- An osteopath is a 'psychologist of the body'. His treatment can help you release emotions through energy shift - somato-emotional response as he sets free the area.

- On the physical side, osteopathy can improve the function of the target area, reduce pain, and bring a better homeostasis to your body. The process may be energy demanding because the body needs to reorganize itself.

- A pain which is too intense can take over the capacity of your brain to focus on essential regulations in your body such as your sleep.

- An osteopathic lesion on the skull, spine or sacrum can disturb the function of the parasympathetic and sympathetic system which controls the stimulation- inhibition of the systems regulating our sleep.

- The osteopath can help the brain change the signal that disturbs the sleep by acting on releasing the tensions that create the pain and by using techniques that regulate the Central Nervous System.

- Listening to your therapist and following his advice is part of the treatment and plays an essential role in your recovery.

"Every day that you open your eyes is a new day and another day to get it right."

JEAN RENEE PORTER, A NEW DAY

CONCLUSION

Sleeping better is not only about sleeping. Feeling better is not only about feeling better. And living better is no only about living better.You need to cook these three ingredients together and in the same kitchen.

Sleeping well depends on how you feel and live. Sleeping better will give you energy and harmony to start the day on the right foot.
Feeling good depends on your mindset, or the perception you have about yourself and life in general. You don't need a reason to be happy. Don't wait to sleep better, live better, get promoted, or win the lottery, to feel good because all of these 'better 'may never happen. You have to be this happy person now instead. It is a state of mind you cultivate everyday. You don't need to find excuses to explain why you are not happy. Mastering your mind and body with self-development concepts and techniques will remind you what is good for you and what is not. You were born to be a winner and to be happy because you deserve it and no one has the right to take this from you. Being happy is your responsibility. You now have the tools to practise.
Living better is a combination of a good night's sleep, a positive state of mind, and good habits. It is essential you understand what you experience in life and how good you are at harmonizing the different aspects of your life all together. You need to pay attention to the details and be in earnest about your desire to get results.

If things happen in life and your answer is to avoid them, the problem will remain. But if you let your 'old-self' behind and open your eyes, you will identify what prevents you from sleeping well, feeling good, and enjoying your life.
Let's imagine for a moment that you are balancing stones in a river... Remember how it feels while doing it. You are at peace and nothing that happens around matters because you are

concentrating on making it look nice, stable, and because it is your moment, it is 'now'. All you need to do is to treat yourself the same way in your life.

Not many people think life is a piece of cake, but a good chef can make miracles happen. So put your hat on and write down your new recipe!

I truly wish this book will help you in your life, in your sleep, with your feelings, and will meet your heart's desire.

Thank you for reading.

INDEX

CONSCIOUS COMPETENCE LADDER OR CONSCIOUS COMPETENCE MATRIX (created by Noel Burch in the 1970s). This illustrates the four stages of learning a skill. The purpose of using the ladder is to identify at what stage of learning a new skill a person is, and the strategies that can be applied for success.
1) Unconsciously unskilled, 2) Consciously unskilled, 3) Consciously skilled, 4) Unconsciously skilled.

CIRCADIAN RHYTHM
This is our internal body clock that regulates the sleep/wake cycles, hormone release, eating habits, etc.

EFT OR EMOTIONAL FREEDOM TECHNIQUE (From Mornah Nalamaku Simeona, Creator Of Self-I-Dentity) is also referred to as 'psychological acupressure'. It consists of releasing emotional blockages from our energy system with non-invasive manual techniques (tip of fingers) targeting the different meridians of the body.

*THE ENERGY THERAPY CENTRE. (n.d. , accessed, 2020, February). *What is EFT? The Origins and Background.* [Blog Post]. Retrieved from http://www.theenergytherapycentre.co.uk/eft-explained.htm

HOMEOSTASIS
The ability to regulate a physiological balance in the body despite external influences from the outside world.

HO'OPONOPONO
"I'm sorry, please forgive me, thank you, I love you", is a Hawaiian prayer, or practice, that consists of forgiving others by clearing any negative energies that link us to them. The technique aims at cutting the connections we have with others that generate stress and negativity, in a loving way. Eventually, "when [we] become right with others, [we] become right with [ourselves]."

* JAMES, M. (2011, May 23, accessed 2020, February). *The Hawaiian Secret of Forgiveness.* [Blog Post]. Retrieved from https://www.psychologytoday.com/intl/blog/focus-forgiveness/201105/the-hawaiian-secret-forgiveness?quicktabs_5=1

* VITALE, J. (n.d, accessed 2020, February). *Transform To Success Your Life With Ho'oponopono. What is Ho'oponopono? And how it helps?* [Blog Post]. Retrieved from
https://joevitalehooponopono.com/success-hooponopono/?gclid=CjwKCAiAvonyBRB7EiwAadauqVlLyEjQfzibKppA1L2votUjtrDzdTgp0NotoMvd9ZEOgFHqG7yDOhoC_i8QAvD_BwE

NEUROTRANSMITTER
A neurotransmitter is a chemical in the brain responsible for neurotransmission. In other words, it allows a message to pass through one cell/neuron to another. Each neurotransmitter has its own function and importance in the brain and body.

NLP
Neuro-Linguistic-Programming is a pseudoscientific and psychological approach that involves the study of our thoughts, language, behaviour and the use of strategies meant to improve our communication skills, change our behaviour and perception of the diverse aspects of life. It is an excellent 'tool' for self-empowerment.

RESTLESS LEGS SYNDROME OR WILLIS-EKBOM DISEASE
This condition can start at any age and tends to get worse over time. It is an 'uncontrollable urge to move your legs' generally during the night.
The discomfort is released with movement.

* MAYO CLINIC. (2020, January 21, accessed 2020, February). *Restless legs syndrome.* [Blog Post]. Retrieved from https://www.mayoclinic.org/diseases-conditions/restless-legs-syndrome/symptoms-causes/syc-20377168

THE LITTLE STICK FIGURES (From Jacques Martel, Author, Trainer, and Speaker).
This is a healing technique, which helps disconnect oneself from emotions that are no longer of any benefit. The purpose is to 'free [one]self from dependencies and attachments involving others in order to bring balance and harmony to our life.

* LES EDITIONS ATMA INTERNATIONALES. (2017, December 3, accessed February 2020). *Jacques Martel Presents The Little Stick Figures Technique In Texas.* [Blog Post]. Retrieved from https://www.atma.ca/en/evenements/jacques-martel-presents-the-little-stick-figures-technique-in-texas/

ACKNOWLEDGTEMENTS

Often in life a few words or pieces of advice coming from a perfect stranger or a dearest friend can resonate with you and bring the strength and power you need to overcome the obstacles you face. These people are your teachers, your challengers and your guardian angels, and I would like to express my sincere gratitude to mine.

With all my heart, I thank my parents for your help, patience, love and understanding. I especially thank my grandfather, Gilbert, whose unconditional love reminds me every day that I am good enough and that whatever I choose to do, I can make it.

To the people I met, and the dear friends I made, during my travels over the last four years. What I have learned from you has positively changed my perception of life. Patricia, Eva, Jimmy, Judy, Sam, Felix, Jasper, David, Safia, Zoé, Élise, Jonathan, Kyra, Neil, Lisa, Rafaela, Bryan, Bella, Ottavia, Shirley, Cheetah, Alex (to name only a few), I thank you for bringing me comfort, confidence and kindness while I was writing this book.

I express special thanks to Pat and Catherine Cocking, to my friends Lisa, Noemi and Bella who kindly helped proofread and edit. Thank you dad for your help and your amazing work on the book cover.

Finally, I thank Gabrielle Bernstein, Gary John Bishop, Rhonda Byrne, Master Sri Akarshana, and many more authors, motivational speakers and influencers. By generously sharing your knowledge, experience and positive vibes with the world through the many books, podcasts and online channels I have read and listened to, you kept me on track when I was doubting myself, and lifted me when I was feeling down.
Thank you all for the peace, kindness, and love I felt during this journey.

BIBLIOGRAPHY

Chapter 2: THE POWER OF A GOOD NIGHT'S SLEEP

1. SLEEP HEALTH FOUNDATION, (2018, Feb 4). *2018 Annual Report.* [PDF File]. Retrieved from https://www.sleephealthfoundation.org.au/files/pdfs/agm/SHF-AnnualReport-260918_WEB.pdf

2. SCOOP MEDIA, (2016, Feb 15). *New study reveals a third of Kiwis are sleep deprived.* [Blog Post]. Retrieved from http://www.scoop.co.nz/stories/BU1602/S00453/new-study-reveals-a-third-of-kiwis-are-sleep-deprived.htm

3. AMERICAN SLEEP APNEA ASSOCIATION, (2017, accessed Aug 2019*). Insufficient sleep is a public health epidemic – CDC.* [Blog Post]. Retrieved from https://www.sleephealth.org/sleep-health/the-state-of-sleephealth-in-america/

4. SOMMEIL.ORG, (Last updated 2020, accessed Sept 2019). *Chiffres et statistiques des troubles du sommeil et de l'insomnie en France.* [Blog Post]. Retrieved from https://www.sommeil.org/comprendre-le-sommeil/chiffres-et-statistiques-des-troubles-du-sommeil-en-france/

5. IO THE INSTITUTE OF OSTEOPATHY, (n.d, accessed Sept 2019). *Sleep Better.* [Blog Post]. Retrieved from https://www.iosteopathy.org/osteopathy-for-health/the-importance-of-sleep/

6. GHOLIPUR, B., (2013, Aug 13, accessed Sept 2019). *Sleeping Pills: Older Adults More Likely to Use.* [LIVE SCIENCE Article]. *Retrieved from* https://www.livescience.com/39278-americans-use-prescription-sleeping-pills.html

7. SLEEP FOUNDATION.ORG, (Last uptaded 2020, accessed Sept 2019). *How Sleep works, The science of sleep- What Happens When You Sleep?* [Article]. Retrieved from https://www.sleepfoundation.org/articles/what-happens-when-you-sleep

8. LUMEN, (n.d, accessed Sept 2019). *Introduction to Psychology – Stages of Sleep.* [Blog Post]. Retrieved from https://courses.lumenlearning.com/wsu-sandbox/chapter/stages-of-sleep/

9. BRANTNER, C. (2019, Feb 2, accessed Sept 2019).*The stages of sleep.* [Blog Post]. Retrieved from https://www.sleepcycle.com/sleep-science/the-stages-of-sleep/

10. Thompson, M. (Last updated 2020, accessed Sept 2019). *How Sleep Works: Neurological Mechanism of Sleep.* [Blog Post]. Retrieved from https://www.howsleepworks.com/how_neurological.html

11. BOWATER, M. (2016, p34-35). *Healing the Nightmare Freeing the Soul.* (1st ed.). Auckland, New Zealand. Calico Publishing Ltd 2016. ISBN 978 1 877429 17 0.

12. BREUS, M. (n.d, accessed Sept 2019). *What is the difference between REM and non REM sleep.* [Blog Post]. Retrieved from https://www.sharecare.com/health/sleep-basics/what-is-nrem-sleep

13. WERBER, B. (2015, p75). *Le sixième sommeil.* (1st ed.). Paris, France. Albin Michel et Bernard Werber Edition. ISBN: 978-2-226-31929-6.

Chapter 3: KEYS TO MEET MR SANDMAN

(1) MAY, J. (n.d, accessed Sept 2019). *"Change: new habits: 'make the familiar unfamiliar': Marisa Peer".* [Blog Post].

Retrieved from https://www.bornfree.space/change-new-habits-make-unfamiliar-familiar-marisa-peer/

(2) Reflection work inspired from the following video.
Master Sri Akarshana. (accessed 2019). Retrieved from Master Sri Akarshana You Tube channel. [Video Files].

(3) BERNETT'S, M. (2019, n32). *Specify Present Situation*. [Video File, accessed via online paid training]. Retrieved from https://www.udemy.com/course/nlp-practitioner-neuro-linguistic-programming-certification-abnlp/learn/lecture/10644830#overview

(4) BISHOP, G, J. (2016, p25-39). *Unfuck Yourself: get out of your head and into your life*. I am willing chapter. (1sr ed.). New York, United States. HarperCollinsPublishers. ISBN: 9780062819499

(5) PROCTOR, Bob. (Last update May 24, 2018, accessed Sept 2019). *Understanding The Power of Paradigms*. [Blog Post]. Retrieved from https://www.proctorgallagherinstitute.com/1974/understanding-the-power-of-paradigms

(6) BK1O1: knowledge Base. (Last update 2020, accessed Sept 2019). *Human Brain. Neuroscience-Cognitive Science*. [Blog Post]. Retrieved from https://www.basicknowledge101.com/subjects/brain.html

(7) PROCTOR, B. (Last update May 24, 2018, accessed Sept 2019). *The Power of Repetition in Shifting a Paradigm*. [Blog Post]. Retrieved from https://www.proctorgallagherinstitute.com/27216/the-power-of-repetition-in-shifting-a-paradigm

(8) KWIK, J. (2019, March 22, accessed Sept 2019). *4 Keys to Changing Your Behavior and Habits*. [Blog Post]. Retrieved from https://jimkwik.com/kwik-brain-101-3-keys-to-changing-your-behavior-habits/

(9) PROCTOR, B. (Last update May 24, 2018, accessed Sept 2019). *Success, Repetition, and Paradigms*. [Blog Post]. Retrieved from https://www.proctorgallagherinstitute.com/39359/success-repetition-and-paradigms.

(10) WATTLES, W. (unknown date, chapter 2). *The Science of Getting Rich.* . [Mobile app. The Law of Attraction].

(11) CARTER, R., ALDRIGE, S., PAGE, M., PARKER, S., FRITH., C., and FRITH., U. (2014, pp. 212-213). *The brain book. (Revised ed.)*. London WC2R ORL, England. Dorling Kindersley Limited. ISBN 978 1 4093 4504 6.

(12) MINDTOOLS TEAM. (n.d, accessed Sept 2019). *The Conscious Competence Ladder*. [Blog Post].Retrieved from https://www.mindtools.com/pages/article/newISS_96.htm

(13) LUDWIG, P., SCHICKER, A. (2018, pp. 101, 102, 108). *End of Procrastination* (2nd ed.). NSW, Australia. Murdoch Books Australia. ISBN 978 1 76063770 5.
(14) BYRNE, R. (2016, p. 7). *The Secret*. (10th ed.). New York, United States. Atria Books. ISBN: 978 1 58270 170 7.

Chapter 5: BASICS AND HABITS

(1) GARNAS, E. (2017, Jun 16, accessed Sept 2019). *It's All Connected*. [Blog Post]. Retrieved from http://darwinian-medicine.com/its-all-connected/

(2) GRABIANOWSKI, E. (n.d., accessed February 2020). *How many skin cells do you shed every day?* [Blog Post]. Retrieved from https://health.howstuffworks.com/skin-care/information/anatomy/shed-skin-cells.htm

(3) LAURIALLO, S. (2019, Jul 9, accessed Sept 2019). *This Is the Best Temperature for Sleeping, According to Experts.* [Blog Post]. Retrieved from https://www.health.com/sleep/best-temperature-for-sleeping

(4) TCHI, R. (2019, Aug 10, accessed Sept 2019). *Feng Shui Tips for Beginners.* [Blog Post]. Retrieved from https://www.thespruce.com/feng-shui-tips-for-beginners-1274536

(5) TOO, L. (2005, pp. 8, n2, n8, …, n26). 168 *Feng Shui ways to a calm and happy life.* (n.s. ed.). London, England. CICO BOOKS Ltd. ISBN: 1 904991 26 2.

(6) SCIENCE LEARNING HUB. POKAPU AKORANGA PUTAIAO. (2007-2020, accessed Sept-Oct 2019). *What is energy?* [Article]. Retrieved from https://www.sciencelearn.org.nz/resources/1572-what-is-energy

(7) TOO, L. (2007, p. 67). *168 Feng Shui Ways to energize your life.* (2nd ed.). New York, United States. CICO BOOKS. ISBN 13: 978 1 904991 95 3/ ISBN 10: 1 904991 95 5.

(8) GAME FROG. (2009, accessed Oct 2019). *Feng Shui Colors.* [Blog Post]. Retrieved from http://chinesehoroscop-e.com/fung-shway/feng-shui-colors.php

(9) TEMMING, M. (2019, Mar 18, accessed Oct 2019). *People can sense Earth's magnetic field, brain waves suggest.* [Blog Post]. Retrieved from https://www.sciencenews.org/article/people-can-sense-earth-magnetic-field-brain-waves-suggest

(10) ABRAMS, A. (2017, Feb 21, accessed Oct 2019). *How Showering at Night Helps You Sleep.* [Blog Post]. Retrieved from https://time.com/4665489/hot-shower-before-bed/

(11) MATEO, A. (Last updated 2018, May 23, accessed Oct 2019). *The Intimate Relationship Between Fitness and Sleep.* [Blog Post]. Retrieved from https://www.everydayhealth.com/fitness/intimate-relationship-between-fitness-sleep/

(12) BERRY, J. (2018, February 6, accessed Sept- Oct 2019). *Endorphins: Effects and how to increase levels.* [Blog Post]. Retrieved from *https://www.medicalnewstoday.com/articles/320839.php*

(13) SLEEP.ORG, NATIONAL SLEEP FOUNDATION. (n.d, 2020, accessed Sept-Oct 2019). *How Exercise Affects Sleep.* [Blog Post]. Retrieved from https://www.sleep.org/articles/exercise-affects-sleep/

(14) CARTER, R., ALDRIGE, S., PAGE, M., PARKER, S., FRITH., C., and FRITH., U. (2014, p. 44). *The brain book.* Body – Brain Size, Energy Use, and Protection. (2nd ed.). London, England. Dorling Kindersley Ltd. ISBN 978 1 4093 4504 6.

(15) DK PUBLISHING. (2010, p. 52) *Everyday Sports Injuries Diagnosis, Treatment, And Prevention* - Concussion sport injuries. (1st ed.) New York, United States. Dorling Kindersley Ltd. ISBN: 978 0 7566 5737 6.

(16) VIOLA SALTZMAN, M, MUSLEH, C. (2016, Feb 15, p.339-348). [Article]. Retrieved from https://www.dovepress.com/traumatic-brain-injury-induced-sleep-disorders-peer-reviewed-fulltext-article-NDT

(17) HELMET.ORG. (2020, Revised statistics Jan 31, accessed Oct 2019 and Feb 2020). *Bicycle Helmet Safety Institute. – Statistics.* [Blog Post]. Retrieved from https://helmets.org/stats.htm

(18) SONNENBURG, J. and E. (2015, May 1, accessed Oct 2019). *Gut Feelings–the "Second Brain" in Our Gastrointestinal Systems [Excerpt] from The Good Gut: Taking Control of Your Weight, Your Mood and Your Long-Term Health.* [Blog Post] Retrieved from https://www.scientificamerican.com/article/gut-feelings-the-second-brain-in-our-gastrointestinal-systems-excerpt/

(19) TUCK SLEEP. (Last update Jul 2019, accessed Oct 2019). *Sleep and Appetite.* [Blog Post] Retrieved from https://www.tuck.com/sleep-and-appetite/

(20) WHITEBREAD, D. (2019, Nov 10, accessed Sept 2019). *Top 10 Foods and Drinks High in Caffeine.* [Blog Post]. Retrieved from https://www.myfooddata.com/articles/high-caffeine-foods-and-drinks.php

(21) TED-Ed. (2017, July 17). *How does caffeine keep us awake? – Hanan Qasim.* [Video File]. Retrieved from https://www.youtube.com/watch?v=foLf5Bi9qXs

(22) BJARNADOTTIR, A. (2017, June 3, accessed Oct 2019). *How Much Caffeine in a Cup of Coffee? A Detailed Guide.* [Blog Post]. Retrieved from https://www.healthline.com/nutrition/how-much-caffeine-in-coffee#section2

(23) MentalHealthDaily (n.d, 2013-19, accessed Oct 2019). *How Long Does It Take For Caffeine To Kick In?* [Blog Post]. Retrieved from https://mentalhealthdaily.com/2018/03/28/how-long-does-it-take-for-caffeine-to-kick-in/

(24) CHERNEY, K. (2018, Nov 6, accessed Sept 2019). *How Long Does Caffeine Stay in Your System?* [Blog Post]. Retrieved from https://www.healthline.com/health/how-long-does-caffeine-last#how-long-symptoms-last

(25) JULSON, E. (2018, May 10, accessed Oct 2019). *10 Best Ways to Increase Dopamine Levels Naturally.* [Blog Post]. Retrieved from https://www.healthline.com/nutrition/how-to-increase-dopamine#section1

(26) KWIK, J. (2019, Jan 4, accessed Oct 2019). *Eating for your brain with Dr. Lisa Mosconi.* [Blog Post].
Retrieved from https://jimkwik.com/kwik-brain-088-eating-for-your-brain-with-dr-lisa-mosconi/

(27) MERCOLA, J. FOOD MATTERS. (2019, November 23). *Top 10 Food Additives to Avoid.* [Blog Post]. Retrieved from https://www.foodmatters.com/article/top-10-food-additives-to-avoid

(28) PEER, M. (2019, March 20, accessed Sept 2019). *Marisa Peer's Rules Of The Mind.* [Blog Post]. Retrieved from https://marisapeer.com/rules-of-the-mind/

(29) BAHL, R. (2018, July 26, accessed Sept 2019). *Even 2 Hours of Dehydration Can Affect Your Body and Brain.* [Blog Post]. Retrieved from https://www.healthline.com/health-news/2-hours-dehydration-can-affect-body-and-brain#1

(30) KHAN, A., MILLER, A., ESPOSITO, L. (2019, July 10, accessed Sept-Oct 2019). *Best Foods for Brain Health.* [Blog Post]. Retrieved from https://health.usnews.com/wellness/food/slideshows/best-foods-for-brain-health

(31) HORMONE HEALTH. (2018, Nov, accessed Oct 2019). *What is Melatonin?* [Blog Post]. Retrieved from https://www.hormone.org/your-health-and-hormones/glands-and-hormones-a-to-z/hormones/melatonin

(32) SLEEPFOUNDATION.ORG. (n.d, 2020, accessed Sept-Oct 2019). *What is Circadian Rhythm?* [Blog Post]. Retrieved from https://www.sleepfoundation.org/articles/what-circadian-rhythm

(33) SCHWARZ, H. (2013, March 5, accessed Oct 2019). *Eating times affect circadian rhythm, study finds.* [Article]. Retrieved from https://yaledailynews.com/blog/2013/03/05/eating-times-affect-circadian-rhythm-study-finds/

(34) SLEEP EDUCATION. AASM. (n.d, 2020, accessed Sept 2019). *Circadian Rhythm Sleep-Wake Disorders.* [Blog Post]. Retrieved from http://sleepeducation.org/sleep-disorders-by-category/circadian-rhythm-disorders

(35) SCACCIA, A. (2019, Aug 13, accessed Sept-Oct 2019). *How to Recognize and Treat the Symptoms of a Nervous Breakdown.* [Blog Post]. Retrieved from https://www.healthline.com/health/mental-26health/nervous-breakdown#symptoms

Chapter 6: YOUR ANCHOR FOR LIFE

(1) PITKO, C. (n.d., 2020, accessed Oct 2019). *An Introduction to Three-Part Yogic Breath.* [Blog Post]. Retrieved from https://www.doyouyoga.com/an-introduction-to-three-part-yogic-breath/

(2) AMERICAN LUNG ASSOCIATION. EDITORAL STAFF. (Last updated 2018, Jun 20, accessed Sept-Oct 2019). *Five Ways You Might Be Breathing Wrong.* [Blog Post] Retrieved from https://www.lung.org/about-us/blog/2018/06/you-might-be-breathing-wrong.html

(3) KEYES, R., Foreword MEHMET C. (2012, p. 39). *The Healing power of Reiki.* (1st ed.). Woodbury Minnesota, United States. Llewellyn publications (Llewellyn Worldwide Ltd). ISBN: 978 0 7387 3351 7.

(4) DALEY, D. (2011, p91). *Exercise to improve your health.* Chapter breathing, Pursed-lip breathing. (n. s. ed.). London, NY. CICO BOOKS. ISBN 978 1907563 69 0

(5) SISSONS, C. (2019, June 25). *What is pursed lip breathing?* [Blog Post- Medical Review]. Retrieved from https://www.medicalnewstoday.com/articles/325555.php

(6) EISLER, M. (2016, January 1). *Learn the Ujjayi Breath, an Ancient Yogic Breathing Technique.* [Blog Post]. Retrieved from https://chopra.com/articles/learn-the-ujjayi-breath-an-ancient-yogic-breathing-technique

Chapter 7: THE ART OF LAUGHING

(1) PINTEREST. Dale Zearfaus profile. (n.d, accessed Oct 2019). [Quote]. Retrieved from https://www.pinterest.com.au/pin/427771664598770264/?lp=true

(2) NEWMAN, T. (2017, January 18, accessed Oct 2019). *Ancient and healthy: The science of laughter.* [Article]. Retrieved from https://www.medicalnewstoday.com/articles/315290.php

(3) ROSEN, D. (2012, May 27, accessed Oct 2019). *Why Laughing In the Evening Helps You Sleep Better at Night.* [Blog Post]. Retrieved from https://www.psychologytoday.com/intl/blog/sleeping-angels/201205/why-laughing-in-the-evening-helps-you-sleep-better-night

(4) WHITEMAN, H. (2017, Jun 3, accessed Oct 2019). *Laughter releases 'fell good hormones; to promote social bonding.* [Article]. Retrieved from https://www.medicalnewstoday.com/articles/317756.php

(5) HEALTHINATION. (Last updated 2018, Jul 5, accessed Sept-Oct 2019). *Wait, Could Laughter Actually Help You Get More Sleep?* [Blog Post]. Retrieved from https://www.healthination.com/health/laughter-improve-sleep

(6) RESEARCHEGATE. (n.d., accessed Oct 2019). *Geriatrics & Gerontology International (Geriatr Gerontol Int).* [Article]. Retrieved from https://www.researchgate.net/journal/1447-0594_Geriatrics_Gerontology_International

(7) SO SOUND SOLUTIONS. (2017, Oct 6, accessed Feb 2019). *Happy Thoughts Benefit Everyone, So Smile.* [Blog Post]. Retrieved from https://www.sosoundsolutions.com/happy-thoughts-benefit-everyone-smile/

Chapter 8: GRATITUDE

(1) HARVARD HEALTH PUBLISHING. HARVARD MEDICAL SCHOOL. (n.d, accessed Oct 2019). *Giving thanks can make you happier.* [Article]. Retrieved from https://www.health.harvard.edu/healthbeat/giving-thanks-can-make-you-happier

(2) CHOWDHURY, M. R. (Last updated 2019, accessed Nov 2019). *The Neuroscience of Gratitude and How It Affects Anxiety and Grief.* [Blog Post]. Retrieved from https://positivepsychology.com/neuroscience-of-gratitude/

(3) ZIVA. ZIVABLOG. (accessed Nov 2019). The neuroscience of gratitude. Blogpost. REetrieved from https://zivameditation.com/zivablog/articles/the-neuroscience-of-gratitude/

(4) CARTER, R., ALDRIGE, S., PAGE, M., PARKER, S., FRITH., C., and FRITH., U. (2014, pp. 72-73). *The brain book. (Revised ed.)* Dorling Kindersley Limited. London WC2R ORL, England. ISBN 978 1 4093 4504 6.

(5) THE HUMAN MEMORY. (2019, Nov 13, accessed Oct2019). *Neurotransmitters and their Functions.* [Blog Post]. Retrieved from https://human-memory.net/neurotransmitters/

(6) EOC INSTITUTE. (n.d, 2020, accessed Oct 2019). *How Meditation Boosts Melatonin, Serotonin, GABA, DHEA, Endorphins, Growth Hormone, & More.* [Blog Post]. Retrieved from https://eocinstitute.org/meditation/dhea_gaba_cortisol_hgh_melatonin_serotonin_endorphins/

(7) LODER, V. (2015, March 18). *How To Rewire Your Brain For Happiness.* [Blog Post]. Retrieved from https://www.forbes.com/sites/vanessaloder/2015/03/18/how-to-rewire-your-brain-for-happiness/#2d054e7d59ef

(8) NOOTROPEDIA. (2016, December 17, accessed Oct 2019). *Braverman Test: How to Understand Your Unique Brain.* [Blog Post]. Retrieved from https://www.nootropedia.com/braverman-test/

Chapter 9: POSITIVE MINDSET

(1) MAY, J. (n.d, accessed Sept 2019). *"Change: new habits: 'make the familiar unfamiliar': Marisa Peer".* [Blog Post]. Retrieved from https://www.bornfree.space/change-new-habits-make-unfamiliar-familiar-marisa-peer/

(2) PEER, M. (2019, Mar 20, accessed Sept 2019). *Marisa Peer's Rules Of The Mind.* [Blog Post]. Retrieved from https://marisapeer.com/rules-of-the-mind/

(3) QUINTERO, N. (2015, March, accessed Oct 2019*). Transforming the mindset: Psychology professor Carol S. Dweck, PhD, speaks at the United Nations.* [Blog Post]. Retrieved from https://www.apa.org/international/pi/2015/03/transforming-mindset

(4) MURPHY, J. (2015). *The Power of your subconscious mind.* Chapter 2: How your own mind works. (n.s. ed). ISBN 10: 8192910962. ISBN 13: 978-8192910963. Amazing Reads.

(5) HAMILTON, D.R. (2014, October 30). *Does your brain distinguish real from imaginary?* [Blog Post]. Retrieved from https://drdavidhamilton.com/does-your-brain-distinguish-real-from-imaginary/

Chapter 10: PLAN TOMORROW

(1) (2) CARMICHAEL, E. (2018, May 26, accessed 2020). 5 Morning ROUTINES That Will TRANSFORM Your LIFE! |
 [Video File]. Retrieved from https://www.youtube.com/watch?v=LmO5aLvwe8A HYPERLINK "https://www.youtube.com/watch?v=LmO5aLvwe8A&index=4&t=0s&list=PLMECJYNZEoysmmdrYgO5MtYfA1eawY8l3" HYPERLINK

(2) Reflection work in part inspired from LUDWIG, P., SCHICKER, A. (2018). *End of Procrastination* (2nd ed.). NSW, Australia. Murdoch Books Australia. ISBN 978 1 76063770 5.

Chapter 11: THE CONDUCTOR OF YOUR NIGHT

(1) HARVARD HEALTH PUBLISHING, HARVARD MEDICAL SCHOOL. (2011, July, accessed Oct 2019). *Music and Health. [Article].* Retrieved from https://www.health.harvard.edu/staying-healthy/music-and-health

(2) SLEEPFOUNDATION.ORG. (n.d, accessed Oct 2019). *Can Music Help You Calm Down and Sleep Better?* [Blog Post]. Retrieved from https://www.sleepfoundation.org/articles/can-music-help-you-calm-down-and-sleep-better

(3) BRAINWORKS TRAIN YOUR MIND. (n.d, accessed Oct 2019). *What are Brainwaves?* [Blog Post]. Retrieved from https://brainworksneurotherapy.com/what-are-brainwaves 201

(4) DISPENZA, J. (2017, Feb 6, accessed Oct 2019). *Playing Your Brain's Symphony: Staying in Tune.* [Blog Post]. Retrieved from https://drjoedispenza.net/blog/general/playing-your-brains-symphony-staying-in-tune/

(5) NCBI. PMC. US NATIONAL LIBRARY OF MEDICINE. NATIONAL INSTITUTES OF HEALTH. (2018, accessed Oct 2019). *The impact of music on the bioelectrical oscillations of the brain.* [Article]. Retrieved from https://www.ncbi.nlm.nih.gov/pmc/articles/PMC6130927/

(6) BREUS, M. (2018, Mar 27, accessed Oct 2019). *Binaural beats: an old sound for better sleep?* [Blog Post]. Retrieved from https://thesleepdoctor.com/2018/03/27/binaural-beats-an-old-sound-for-better-sleep/

(7) THE WELLNESS ENTREPRISE. (2017, Mar 23, accessed Dec 2019). Dr. Masaru Emoto and Water Consciousness. [Blog Post]. Retrieved from https://thewellnessenterprise.com/emoto/

(8) MURPHY, J. (2015). *The Power of your subconscious mind.* Chapter 2: How your own mind works. ISBN 10: 8192910962. ISBN 13: 978-8192910963. Amazing Reads.

Chapter 12 : THE POWER OF NATURE

(1) HOUDRET, J. (2012, pp. 30-31*). Herbal Teas And Heath infusions.* Teas For Calm And Sleep. (n.s. ed.). Leicestershire, England. LORENZ BOOKS. ISBN-10: 0754821722. ISBN-13: 978-0754821724.

(2) INDIGO HERBS OF GLASTONBURY SINCE 2004. (n.d, accessed Sept 2019). *Vervain Benefits.* [Blog Post]. Retrieved from https://www.indigo-herbs.co.uk/natural-health-guide/benefits/vervain

(3) RAMOS, M. (2018, Aug 15, accessed Oct 2019). *Top 5 Single-Plant Sleep Remedies.* [Blog Post]. Retrieved from https://goodnights.rest/bed-botany-and-beyond/5-single-plant-sleep-remedies/

(4) SERRAS, L. (2019, Jul 12, accessed Oct 2019). *15 Scents to Help You Sleep.* [Blog Post]. Retrieved from https://www.fragrancex.com/blog/scents-to-help-you-sleep/

(5) EASON, C. (2013, pp. 8, 15). *Crystals for love and relationships.* (Revised ed. 2010, originally published in the New Crystal Bible). London, England. CARLTON BOOKS. ISBN: 978 1 78097 452 1.

(6) RADFORD, B. (2013, Feb 21, accessed Sept 2019). *Why Is Quartz Used in Watches?* [Blog Post]. Retrieved from https://www.livescience.com/32509-why-is-quartz-used-in-watches.html

(7) BROWN, D. (2019, pp. 43, 108-109, 133-134, 170). *Crystal bliss.* Attract Love. Feed Your Spirit. Manifest Your Dreams. (Reprint edition). Massachusetts, United States. ADAMS MEDIA. ISBN-10: 1721400141. ISBN-13: 978-1721400140.

(8) PAULIN, J. Y. (2012, p. 84). *La Mystique Des Pierres.* (revised edition, 1st ed. in 2002). India. White Sadhu Publishers. ISBN: 978 2 917369 01 2.

(9) INSURANCE INFORMATION INSTITUTE. (n.d, accessed Sept- Oct 2019). *Facts + Statistics: Pet statistics.* [Blog Post].
Retrieved from https://www.iii.org/fact-statistic/facts-statistics-pet-statistics

(10) FELLIWAY. (2018, Jan 8, accessed Oct 2019). *7 Reasons Why Humans & Cats Are A Match Made In Heaven.* [Blog Post]. Retrieved from https://medium.com/chilled-cat/7-reasons-why-humans-cats-are-a-match-made-in-heaven-cea37ad9fc24

(11) SILVER, J. (n.d., accessed Oct 2019). *Letting Your Cat Purr On Your Body Can Have A Huge Impact On Your Health.* [Blog Post]. Retrieved from https://www.littlethings.com/benefits-of-cat-purrs

(12) DOWLING, S. (2018, Jul 25, accessed Feb 2020). *The complicated truth about a cat's purr.* [Article]. Retrieved from https://www.bbc.com/future/article/20180724-the-complicated-truth-about-a-cats-purr

Chapter 13 MEDITATION

(1) RAKICEVIC, M. (2019, Jul 12, accessed Nov 2010). *27 Meditation Statistics That You Should Be Aware Of.* [Blog Post].
Retrieved from https://disturbmenot.co/meditation-statistics/

(2) MASTER SRI AKARSHANA. (2019, February 15, accessed 2019). *Himalayan Yogi Reveals How to Meditate Properly | The Secret [MUST WATCH!!].* [Video File]. Retrieved from https://www.youtube.com/watch?v=3ST5M-HXSrU

(3) SHEA, M., DILLARD-WRIGHT, D. B. AND JERATH, R. (2011, p. 2). *The Everything guide to meditation for healthy living.* Section to meditate or not meditate. (n.s. ed.). Avon, Massachussets. Adamsmedia.

(4) MASTER SRI AKARSHANA. (2018, Jun 25, accessed 2019). *How to meditate properly. | Lessons From a Yogi Master [Most People Get This Wrong!!].* [Video File]. Retrieved from https://www.youtube.com/watch?v=i7kaS8MkSr0

(5) BERNARD BECKWITH, R. M., BUTERA, R., MIKULAS, W. L., BYRON, E., SCHER., A. B., PARK, K., ... KHALSA., S. (2016, p. 9). *Complete Book Of Mindful.* The mind in mindfulness meditation. (1st ed.). LLEWELLYN Publications. Woodbury, MN, United States. ISBN: 9780738746777 and 9780738750835.

(6) SHEA, M., DILLARD-WRIGHT, D. B. AND JERATH, R. (2011, p. 199-200). *The Everything guide to meditation for healthy living*. Chapter 16. Meditative Toning. (n.s. ed.). Avon, Massachussets. Adamsmedia.

(7) MINDWORKS. (2020, Jan 30, accessed Oct 2019). *What are the Different Types of Meditation?* [Blog Post]. Retrieved from https://mindworks.org/blog/different-types-meditation-technique/

(8) DISPENZA, J. (2017, Feb 6, accessed Oct 2019). *Playing Your Brain's Symphony: Staying in Tune*. [Blog Post]. Retrieved from https://drjoedispenza.net/blog/general/playing-your-brains-symphony-staying-in-tune/

(9) EOC INSTITUTE. (n.d., accessed Oct 2019). *How Meditation Boosts Melatonin, Serotonin, GABA, DHEA, Endorphins, Growth Hormone, & More*. [Article]. Retrieved from https://eocinstitute.org/meditation/dhea_gaba_cortisol_hgh_melatonin_serotonin_endorphins/

(10) EOC INSTITUTE. (n.d., accessed Oct 2019). *Harnessing Neuroplasticity: 9 Key Brain Regions Upgraded Through Meditation*. [Article]. Retrieved from https://eocinstitute.org/meditation/10-key-brain-regions-upgraded-with-meditation-2/#codeword1

(11) CARTER, R., ALDRIGE, S., PAGE, M., PARKER, S., FRITH., C., and FRITH., U. (2014, p. 187). *The brain book*. Body –Altering Consciousness. (2nd ed.). London, England. Dorling Kindersley Ltd. ISBN 978 1 4093 4504 6.

(12) EOC INSTITUTE. (n.d., accessed Oct 2019). *How Brainwave Entrainment With EquiSync® Can Change Your Life.* [Article]. Retrieved from https://eocinstitute.org/meditation/brainwave_charts_brainwave_patterns/

(13) MASTER SRI AKARSHANA. (2017, July 1, accessed 2019). *How to Calm Your Mind Without Sitting to Meditate.* [Video File]. Retrieved from https://www.youtube.com/watch?v=60pBM9xR19s

Chapter 14 : DREAMS

(1) BOWATER, M. (2016, p. 43). *Healing the Nightmare Freeing the Soul*. (n.s. ed.). Auckland, New Zealand. Calico publications. ISBN 978 1 877429 17 0.

(2) CARTER, R., ALDRIGE, S., PAGE, M., PARKER, S., FRITH., C., and FRITH., U. (2014, p. 161). *The brain book*. Laying down a memory. (2nd ed.). London, England. Dorling Kindersley Ltd. ISBN 978 1 4093 4504 6.

(3) NIH. NATIONAL INSTITUTES OF HEALTH. (2019, Sep 20, accessed Jan 2020). *The brain may actively forget during dream sleep.* [Article]. Retrieved from https://www.nih.gov/news-events/news-releases/brain-may-actively-forget-during-dream-sleep

(4) CARTER, R., ALDRIGE, S., PAGE, M., PARKER, S., FRITH., C., and FRITH., U. (2014, p. 189). *The brain book*. Body – Sleep and Dreams. (2nd ed.). London, England. Dorling Kindersley Ltd. ISBN 978 1 4093 4504 6.

(5), (6) BOWATER, M. (2016, p. 32, 43). *Healing the Nightmare Freeing the Soul*. (n.s. ed.). Auckland, New Zealand. Calico publications. ISBN 978 1 877429 17 0.

(7) SLEEPFOUNDATION.ORG. (n.d., accessed Jan 2020). *How Alcohol Affects the Quality—And Quantity—Of Sleep*. [Article]. Retrieved from https://www.sleepfoundation.org/articles/how-alcohol-affects-quality-and-quantity-sleep

(8) GOYAL, S., KAUSHAL, J., GUPTA, MC., VERMA, S. (2013, Mar 10, accessed Jan 2020) *Drugs and Dreams*. [PDF File] Retrieved from http://medind.nic.in/iaa/t13/i3/iaat13i3p624.pdf

(9), (10) BOWATER, M. (2016, pp. 95, 22-34). *Healing the Nightmare Freeing the Soul*. (n.s. ed.). Auckland, New Zealand. Calico publications. ISBN 978 1 877429 17 0.

(11) MACMILLAN, A. (2017, Oct 27, accessed Jan 2020). *Why Dreaming May Be Important for Your Health*. [Blog Post]. Retrieved from https://time.com/4970767/rem-sleep-dreams-health/

Chapter 15: THE BEAUTY OF REIKI

(1) KEYES, R., Foreword MEHMET C. (2012). *The Healing power of Reiki*. Chapter What Reiki is. (1st ed.). Woodbury Minnesota, United States. Llewellyn publications (Llewellyn Worldwide Ltd). ISBN: 978 0 7387 3351 7.

(2) CAMPION, L. Foreword by THOMAS, R. (2018, p. 3). *The art of psychic Reiki*. Introduction-Reiki and healing (n.s. ed). Oakland, CA, United States. Reveal press. ISBN10 1684031214 and ISBN13 9781684031214.

(3) GREEN LOTUS. (2011, accessed Oct 2019). *Reiki Really Works: A Groundbreaking Scientific Study*. [PDF File]. Retrieved from https://www.uclahealth.org/rehab/workfiles/urban%20zen/research%20articles/reiki_really_works-a_groundbreaking_scientific_study.pdf

(4) DORAN, B. (2009, accessed Oct 2019). *The Science Behind Reiki*. [PDF File - Article]. Retrieved from https://www.equilibrium-e3.com/images/PDF/Science%20Behind%20Reiki.pdf

Chapter 16 : OSTEOPATHY

(1) PAYROUSE, J.L. (2010-2011). *Osteopathie et Medecine*. [PDF File from CENTRE DOSTEOPATHIE ATMAN – OSTEOPATHIE ET MEDECINE- 2010-2011– GLOSSAIRE-PHILOP1ATMAN]. From osteopathic teachings.

(2) BOZZETTO, M. (2010-2011, p. 55). *Osteopathie et Medecine*. [PDF File from CENTRE DOSTEOPATHIE ATMAN – OSTEOPATHIE ET MEDECINE- 2010-2011–HISTOIRE OSTEOPATHIE]. From osteopathic teachings.

(3) FRYMANN, V.M. (n.d. accessed Nov 2019). *The Philosophy of Osteopathy*. [Article]. Retrieved from http://www.somatherapy.info/Osteopathy.html

(4) LIEN MECANIQUE OSTEOPATHIQUE. (Last updated 2020, accessed Oct 2019). *More about Mechanical Link*. [Online]. Retrieved from https://lmosteo.com/en/more-about-mechanical-link

(5) NCBI. PNAS authors. (2013, Dec 30, accessed Oct 2019). *Bodily Maps of Emotions*. [Article]. Retrieved from https://www.ncbi.nlm.nih.gov/pmc/articles/PMC3896150/

(6) TEYCHENE, C. (2017, Mar 1, accessed Oct 2019). *Osteopathy for sleep disorders*. [Blog Post]. Retrieved from https://un-osteo.com/osteopathy-sleep-disorders/

(7) RHEAULT, L. (2018, Jan 1, accessed Oct 2019). *The Effectiveness of Osteopathy on Insomnia*. [Blog Post]. Retrieved from https://connecthealthcare.ca/effectiveness-osteopathy-insomnia/

SHORT STORY OF THE BOOK

This book was written while traveling in 2019. It has been my dearest companion in Australia, Fiji Islands, New Zealand, The Philippines, Taiwan, Thailand, England and France.

The photos were taken in New Zealand.

"The World is your Oyster"
WILLIAM SHAKESPEARE

Printed in Great Britain
by Amazon